Collins

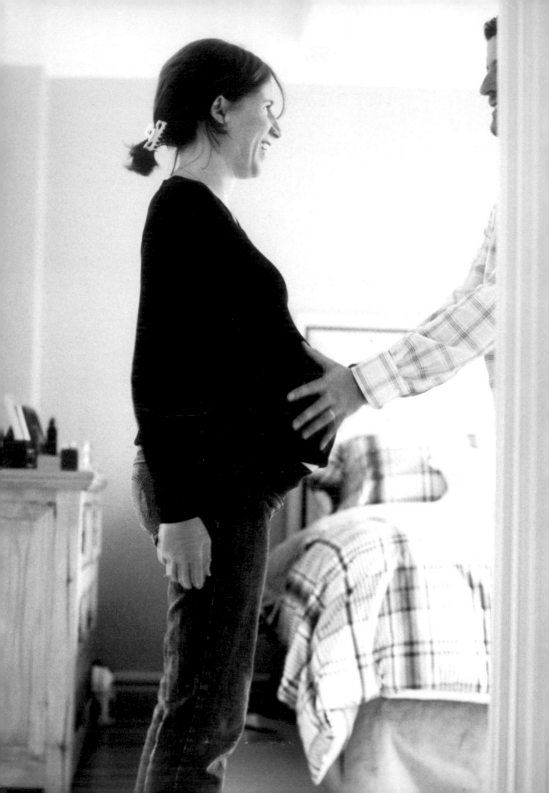

need to know?

Pregnancy

Harriet Sharkey

Collins

I dedicate this book to my children, Patrick and Rosa, and to Dee, my partner in adventure. You light up my life.

First published in 2006 by Collins
an imprint of
HarperCollins Publishers
77–85 Fulham Palace Road
London W6 8JB

www.collins.co.uk

09   08   07   06
5   4   3   2   1

A catalogue record for this book is available from the British Library

Editor: Emma Callery
Designer: Bob Vickers
Picture research: Laura Kesner
Illustrator: Amanda Williams
Series design: Mark Thomson
Front cover photograph © Gusto Images/Getty Images
Back cover photographs © Bubbles, bottom picture © Versha Jones

ISBN-10 0-00-721334-4
ISBN-13 978-0-00-721334-4

Colour reproduction by by Colourscan, Singapore
Printed and bound by by Printing Fxpress, Hong Kong

The quotation on page 41 appears with kind permission of Clairview Books. It is taken from *Birth and Breastfeeding* by Michael Odent (published 2003, ISBN 1 902636 48 1).

Picture credits
p.1, 6 © Glenn Glasser/zefa/Corbis; p.9 © Larry Williams/Corbis; p.10, 142, 165 © Owen Franken/Corbis; p.13, 55, 160 © Dumas/Mediscan; p.15, 150, 152 © Harriet Sharkey; p.17, 60, 85 © Bubbles/Chris Rout; p.21, 25, 37, 83 © H. Schmid/zefa/Corbis; p.27 © Lawrence Manning/Corbis; p.29 © Eddie Lawrence/Mother & Baby Picture Library; p.31 © Ariel Skelley/Corbis; p.57, 77, 78 © Bubbles/Moose Azim; p.32, 133, 161 © Bubbles/Frans Rombout; p.40 © Caterina Bernardi/zefa/Corbis; p.45 © Ian Hooton/Mother & Baby Picture Library; p.50 © Jim Craigmyle/Corbis; p.63 © Dennis Wilson/Corbis; p.67, 118, 129 © Greenhill/Mediscan; p.71, 72, 88 © Clinical Diagnostic Services, London; p.87 © Brigitte Sporrer/zefa/Corbis; p.90 © LWA-Dann Tardif/Corbis; p.96, 117 © Bubbles/Loisjoy Thurstun; p.97 © Franco Vogt/Corbis; p.99, 114 © Bubbles/Jennie Woodcock; p.101 © Steve Prezant/Corbis; p.110, 125, 134, 154 © Ben Cowlin; p.123, 137 © Bubbles/Angela Hampton; p.131 © Moose Azim/Mother & Baby Picture Library; p.140 © Jules Perrier/Corbis; p.145 © Rob Huibers/Panos Pictures; p.148 © Sven Torfinn/Panos Pictures; p.157 © Patricia McDonough/Corbis; p.164 © Versha Jones; p.166 © Martin Harvey/Corbis.

Contents

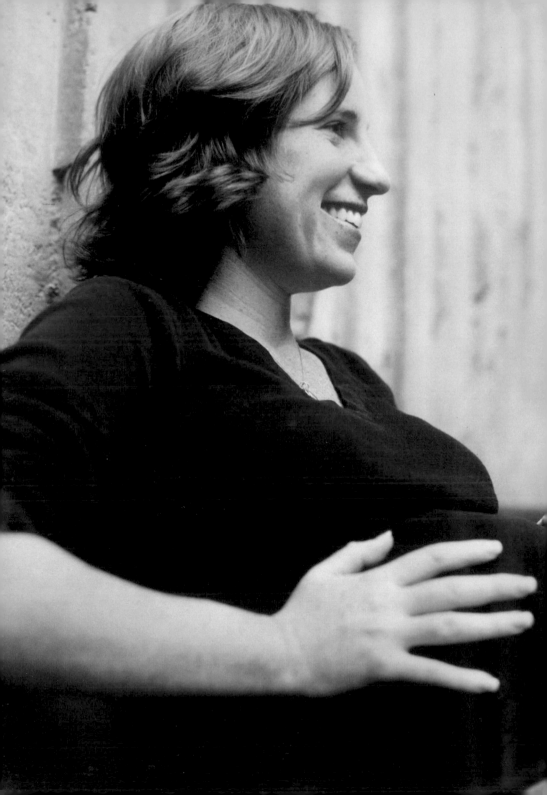

1 Being pregnant

There can be no generalizations about pregnancy – every person's experience is unique, and while one woman may feel tired and low, another is bouncing around with more energy than she has ever had. It's the same with labour: one person may be beset with problems, another apparently 'breeze' through it. This book is not about what pregnancy *should* be, because there is no such thing. It is a guide through the weeks and months, intended to answer your questions ...

'The journey into parenthood is one of the most exciting transitions and times in your life. It is a wonderful opportunity to explore who you are so that you can open yourself to welcoming your new baby. Many men and women say that their children teach them so much. Enjoy the exploration.'
Dr Yehudi Gordon

So you're pregnant

Ecstatic, shocked, numb, surprised, pleased, unsure ... all these are common reactions to the confirmation of pregnancy. In a moment of truth, life changes completely. There is another person in your life and he – or she – is already dependent on you.

A good start in life

The idea of being responsible can be unnerving, but it is good to know that your body is prepared to nurture this life, to give birth, and to mother. A man, too, is genetically primed to be a father. This is nature's most basic intent, and nature is always there to help you. Even so, you may need to make changes to create the best possible pregnancy environment for you and your baby. You may also need some effort – and courage – to accept the changes that are happening to you.

There are three crucial elements to pregnancy. The first is your baby – what kind of life will she have in the womb, and how will she enter the world and be welcomed? The second is you – how you feel, and how you nurture yourself and your relationship. The third is birth. How will you prepare to realise your dreams and help your baby through a peaceful transition, and to adjust if things don't go as you expect?

Your baby

Science, religion, folklore and mythology do not between them have the answer to life – what it is that makes each baby such a charismatic, engaging and unique person. There are suspicions and anecdotes as well as scientifically proven facts, however, that reveal how important pregnancy is for a baby's physical and emotional wellbeing. Your baby is your passenger, and while you cannot take full responsibility for her development or character, you can take steps to create the best possible environment for her to thrive and to prepare for life beyond the womb. Changes that take place naturally during pregnancy help you to do this.

You

In nine months you may feel more emotions than you thought possible. This is as true for a man as it is for a woman, although a woman is more likely to be carried by unpredictable emotional tides.

All your feelings, however light, dark, crazy or confusing, are important, hormonally influenced or otherwise. Not only does pregnancy mark the threshold of a hugely significant change in your life, it also opens you to emotional aspects of yourself that may have been hidden for years, even since your own childhood. Physical changes, altered sleep patterns and dreams encourage emotions to surface into your unconscious or conscious mind. Sometimes this is exciting, amazing even; sometimes it is confronting and difficult to integrate.

The myth that pregnant women feel constantly happy is reality for some people. Indeed, this may be the best time of your life. If it's not, you may be reassured to know that this is normal too. If negative feelings continue, do confide in someone you trust. Expressing your emotions with someone you trust could help to improve your experience of pregnancy and your confidence. It may be more valuable now than at any other time of your life.

Even in early pregnancy your baby has a powerful presence.

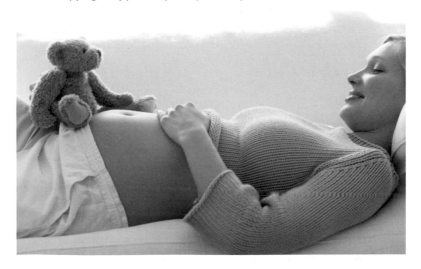

**Find out what you can about
birth, and beyond ...
knowledge is power.**

Gifts for life

Although you cannot control everything, you may
want to make some commitments that could
enhance your journey through pregnancy and birth.
The first is to trust yourself and your baby, who
instinctively knows how to grow and thrive. This is
not to say you do not need companionship, however.
The journey is new and if you have a network of
friends, family and healthcare professionals, they
will help you on the way. Building a team of people
who will be there for you is the single greatest gift
you can offer yourself.

The second gift is to be informed. You don't need
to become an expert but it will help to have some
awareness of what lies ahead. Dare to look beyond

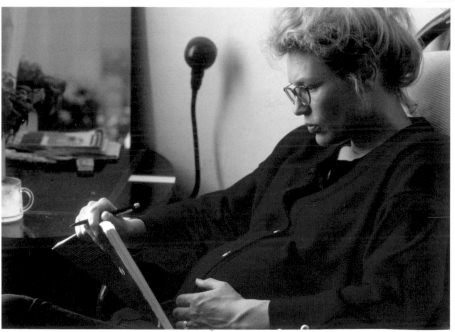

pregnancy too. The more you know, the better prepared you will be.

The third gift involves your partnership: give it attention, time and space. You may find that your intimacy increases; but at the same time tensions and niggles can grow, and when your baby is with you the quality of your relationship will change. Pregnancy provides an opportunity to work through issues of conflict and to share your hopes and fears. If you clear some cobwebs and prepare strong foundations, it will be easier to weather changes in the future. If you are not with your baby's father, it may still be important to maintain your relationship.

Birth

In a first pregnancy, birth is a mystery, an event in the future shrouded in hope and uncertainty. Even in subsequent pregnancies birth is unpredictable. Birth may be the most amazing event in your life and a gentle welcome for your baby. At the other end of the spectrum, birth may turn out to be a frightening or shocking experience. Part of your focus in pregnancy will be preparing for birth and you will find plenty of advice on pages 112-47.

It is a challenge to marry medical knowledge and skill with traditional wisdom and loving support. This winning combination is becoming a reality in a number of birth centres across the world, but it is not always in place. In some hospitals, women talk of being uninformed, left alone and dehumanized even. This sad but true situation is not universal, but you do have a say in your first choice of birth location, and your preparations could make a difference for you and for your baby.

Here comes dad

There are an infinite number of wonderful aspects to becoming a father and many men are surprised how easily they adapt. There will also be challenges as you get used to things. Your peers who are dads will probably tell you this, quite possibly with a dose of cynicism and something along the lines of, 'Just you wait!'

Change for the better?

What you're waiting for, according to your cynical mates, may be broken sleep, the challenge of soothing your crying baby, anxiety about her wellbeing, mopping up your partner's tears, and getting used to only one night out a month (or even less). But to focus on just this would be to play down what is probably the most amazing part of any man's life.

If you are happy and excited, you'll probably love your journey into parenthood. What's more, your partner will know that you are on side, and your baby will feel loved and welcomed. It's a good recipe for enjoying fatherhood and enriching your family. On the other hand, if you are nervous or unhappy, things will be different, whether you share your feelings or keep your cards close to your chest.

'My advice is, take it in your stride. Be confident. That's all you can do. Your life is going to be different but things won't be totally, 100% parenthood. You can keep part of what you know, like you can take your baby to the pub for a pint with your wife or partner, not all the time, but you can.'
Tim, father of two

What you can do

The most valuable thing you can do is to learn about pregnancy and birth – from this and other books, including some aimed exclusively at dads, and from your partner and maybe from classes. Knowledge is power – for you and for your partner with whom you're sharing this journey.

While your partner is in touch with your baby – literally – throughout

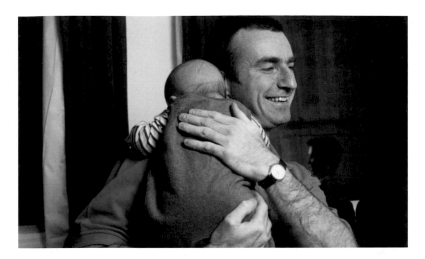

pregnancy, and has hormones to help her feel loving and nurturing, you are only able to stand by and sympathize. This huge physiological difference, although obvious, can be ignored and some men feel criticized for not being involved or excited 'enough' even though they are doing their best. Talking to your partner about the way you feel, even though this may be scary, is preferable to bottling it up. As you listen to one another you may both feel better. You can also get closer: your baby hears you speak and will recognize your voice when you meet after birth. She can also feel you stroking and massaging her through your partner's abdomen.

After the birth, spending time with your baby will help you to get in touch with one another: the effect will be most dramatic if you rest together, skin to skin. Your breathing rhythms, heartbeats and temperatures will become synchronized as you feel and smell one another. This is a winning recipe for bonding, particularly if you have felt out of touch during pregnancy.

For more information, see *Dads: Because Bringing Up Kids Ain't Hard* by Mal Peachey and *Fatherhood: The Truth* by Marcus Berkmann.

'My dad wasn't there when I was a baby, and died when I was 12. I've no idea what to do. Sally will do it all. Won't she?'
James

Relationships

Before babies, it's just you. Having a tiny and dependent person in your life is quite different. And whatever you choose to imagine before the birth, nothing can prepare you for reality – either the depth of feeling or the change to your own patterns of sleeping, eating, washing or socializing. You may adapt easily.

You and your partner

If you're in a relationship, the way you adapt will reflect whether you are going into parenthood as a team, or as two individuals. There is no right or wrong, but you can gather a few tools that could help you both enjoy family life, and provide security and loving guidance for your child.

You each come from different families with different ideas about childcare, eating and even communicating. Unwittingly, you each react to your backgrounds – either you'll repeat them or try to do the opposite. A lot depends on your experiences as children. You may not always be in agreement. Talking about your views (which may involve sleeping arrangements, naming, breastfeeding, working, where to live, and more) will be useful. If you discover differences of opinion before your baby is born, you may be able to come to a happy compromise in advance, or seek further advice if you can't agree. Understanding and mutual support are like golden tickets in any relationship when babies come along. Take time to talk and to be together.

Pregnant without a partner

If you are pregnant and single, you may not be concerned about culture clashes and working as a team with your baby's father. For more on what you may face as a single parent, dip into *Going It Alone* by Natascha Mirosch.

You and your baby

Your baby's emotional learning is intense and you can help her to feel respected, contented and acknowledged. If you are inclined to 'manage' your baby, you may perceive her as a foreign body growing inside you, following a process in which you are not involved. If you are a 'nurturer', you'll feel you are actively growing your baby and there is communication between you. After birth, you may adapt to your baby (nurturing) or expect your baby to adapt to you (managing).

These are, of course, stereotypes and you probably fall somewhere in between. Perhaps your feelings will change through pregnancy or after birth. From a baby's point of view, it is better to be nurtured than managed. The term 'managed' is also applied to labour when obstetric decisions can take precedence over a woman's instincts and preferences, leaving a woman feeling ignored, disrespected and angry or dejected. A baby who feels managed may have the same reaction. On the other hand, feeling nurtured is likely to make a baby feel good, so that she delights in expressing herself, exploring and learning. This is a wonderful foundation for her.

The period of babyhood is one of the most beautiful and precious times of human life, both for babies and for the adults who nurture them. From conception, life has already begun. Pregnancy marks the beginning of what will probably be the most significant relationship, and the greatest adventure, you will ever have.

Being pregnant 'together' is part of your journey as a couple and a family.

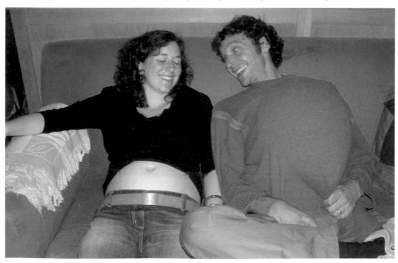

Hopes and reality

Pregnancy is a time of expectations. It is important to have a vision that inspires you, and help you make a stand for what matters to you. Acknowledging your hopes – and reality – will help you create a positive environment for pregnancy and birth.

Your expectations

Try completing the following sentences. Your hopes may change from month to month.

▶ In pregnancy, I wish for ...
▶ I think I will feel ...
▶ My image of birth is ...
▶ I expect my partner to ...
▶ I expect my baby to ...
▶ I expect my family and friends to ...
▶ I expect parenthood to be ...

Some things may not go as you wish. Surprises may involve your physical health, your emotions, your partner, your finances, your choice of hospital, your baby's behaviour ... and more.

The difference between what's planned and what actually happens is not necessarily a problem. You may dream of giving birth in water and end up on dry land; imagine using an epidural and on the day rely on your breath; plan to avoid all pain relief and end up using several methods and being very pleased you did. You might dream of bliss, but feel blue. If you are upset, angry or disappointed, it helps to acknowledge this, and to talk about it. For support, look to your family and friends, your birth team, books and websites, your faith and your baby.

Positive planning

▶ Make a note of your preferences, particularly concerning the environment for birth.
▶ Visualize your hopes now and then, or as often as each day (page 91).

▶ Invite your body and your baby to prepare for birth. This is beneficial for a vaginal birth and a caesarean.

▶ Be aware that things may not go according to plan. Keep an open mind and remember that you, your baby and your partner influence the dynamic.

▶ If you cannot accept the reality or you are frightened, talk to someone you trust. Consider visiting a professional counsellor.

Managing your time

While you are pregnant, the way you divide your time may carry on relatively unchanged. But if you are tired, if you wish to spend more time exercising or need to fit in antenatal appointments, you may need to shuffle things around. Organizing your days and weeks to relieve pressure on yourself and create time to be with your partner, your parents and others is good practice for time management once your baby is born.

▶ Don't aim to do everything in one day. Space your commitments and ask for help to ease your load.

▶ There may be ways to ease pressure at work.

▶ Allow time each day to relax – even ten minutes can work wonders (see page 30).

▶ Allow time to shop and cook food that is nourishing (see pages 20–5).

▶ Create time to exercise: at least 20 minutes a day and always appropriate to your stage of pregnancy (see pages 28–31).

▶ Give yourself permission to slow down, particularly in early pregnancy when you may be very tired.

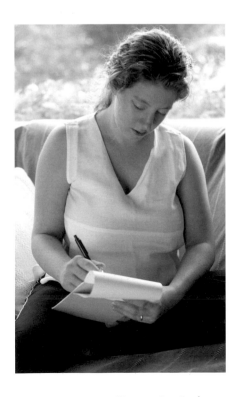

Keeping a journal is a record of your once-in-a-lifetime journey

Money and work

Finances can be a thorny issue and increase feelings of pressure, particularly if maternity and paternity leave involve a drop in income, or you wish to fund private medical care or help at home.

As society emerges from a 'doing it all' culture men and women are admitting that trying to do everything is not always for the best. It is a challenge to continue a full-time career *and* nurture relationships at home *and* feel calm. You may need to sit down and work out what is more important in your baby's early years: money or time?

Will you (both) continue to work? Can one of you go part time? Do you need to apply for benefits? Do you plan to use childcare? Do you want a career change? You do not have to solve everything but simply bringing up important issues could reduce anxiety and make practical decisions easier later on (see also pages 32–3).

The stress factor

It is completely normal for expectant mums and dads to feel anxious now and then, particularly if there are medical concerns or difficulties around money, housing, work or relationships. Mild anxiety may prompt you to find out more or discuss what's bothering you. It's a good thing in moderation, and won't harm your baby.

There is evidence, however, that when maternal stress levels are high babies often follow suit (with greatest effect if mum is very stressed in the third trimester of pregnancy). Not all babies are adversely affected but potential consequences include lower birth weight, difficulty in labour, irritability and restlessness after birth, and a tendency to stress in later life.

Anxiety arises because of what's happening in your life and because of the way you perceive and react to the situation. Many events are beyond your control and your coping mechanisms may be similarly difficult to control: you have unconscious habits and while some are helpful, others

The ABC

A

Ask what's happening	You may need to seek a second opinion
Ask for help to improve the way you feel	Help can be practical, medical or complementary

B

Be kind to yourself	Try things that could make you feel better. Eat well, exercise and rest. You might also benefit from some pampering

C

Communicate the way you feel to the people who are important in your life, and to your healthcare team	This may involve looking at difficult issues, perhaps problems in relationships or previous experiences that trouble you. Some people find it really helpful to be in touch with other parents or expectant parents
Communicate with your baby too	Tell her what is happening, what you feel, and that any anxiety is not her fault. It makes the experience lighter for you and many brain and behavioural scientists believe blame-free communication is a great foundation for a good relationship and for a baby's sense of self-worth in years to come

may increase your anxiety. If you are stressed, initial changes to your hormones, nerves, muscles and thoughts will help you cope but if they are prolonged they may provoke further anxiety and a cycle may set in. The ABC (see box above) may help you relieve anxiety before this cycle begins, or gradually move away from long-term stress.

Some people find it helps to look more closely at stress: apparently obvious factors may be symptoms of something deeper. For instance, you may be spending extra time at work (the stressful factor) as a way of avoiding uncomfortable feelings at home (the cause). If something from your past is troubling you, professional support may be really beneficial.

Food focus

You are what you eat and so, therefore, is your baby. In pregnancy, when your sensations of taste and smell enter new realms and you become more keenly aware of your body, you have a wonderful opportunity to take a fresh look at food.

Eating for health

The most basic thing you need to know is that the more natural the food you eat, the better. The second important guideline is to eat a moderately sized and balanced meal every three to four hours. Even if you forget the detail, remembering these two fundamentals will make it easier to eat well and feel good for the rest of your life.

Feeling up to it?

If you're finding it difficult to eat well, there may be practical reasons but, in all probability, there will also be an emotional element. To eat is to nourish yourself, and how you do this reflects your self-esteem and your feelings. If you feel anxious or devalued, for instance, your instinct may be to say, 'To hell with it.' It's easy, in fact, to get caught in a cycle where what you eat makes you feel bad, and feeling bad triggers cravings for the same food again.

Eating well can soon improve your mood and your body image, yet breaking a negative cycle might take a lot of courage and commitment. It will be easier if you feel encouraged and have someone with whom you can cook and eat.

Try taking note of how you feel if you reach for food that isn't good for you, eat when you are not hungry or deny yourself food. Does this shift an uncomfortable feeling? What happens emotionally and to your body after a day or two of balanced eating? Eating well really does give an energy buzz and has so many benefits – you deserve to be lovingly nurtured and so does your baby. Enjoying food in company will boost the feel-good hormones flowing through your body and to your baby.

Energy food and the sugar trap

You get energy from natural sugars in food. The energy release may be strong but short lived or it may be gradual. It's best to have a basis of foods that release their energy slowly – complex carbohydrates accompanied by whole foods.

Foods that release sugar quickly don't give you energy for long. These include processed and refined foods – sweets and chocolates, cakes, croissants and biscuits – as well as concentrated fruit juice

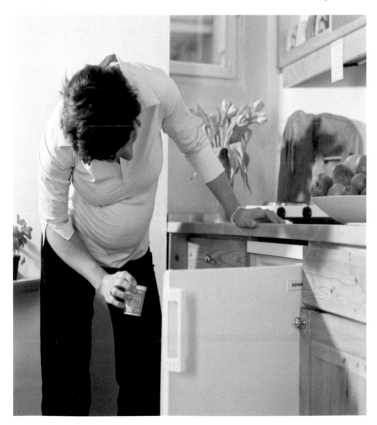

With a good supply of fresh fruit and healthy snacks you won't go hungry, and may be less tempted to reach for the chocolate.

good to know

Chilling down
Some foods help to reduce anxiety by calming your nervous system. Try garlic, which also reduces high blood pressure, and oats, which are delicious soaked in water or soya milk, topped with cut fruit and nuts.

without pulp, many ready-made meals and sugary hot and cold drinks. Your blood sugar levels rise quickly, but then fall drastically, the resulting hypoglycaemia (low blood sugar) causes feelings including restlessness, faintness, anxiety, paranoia, moodiness, hunger and nausea for you and for your baby. It also disturbs hormone balance. You can avoid hypoglycaemia by eating good food every three to four hours.

The measure of energy potential is sometimes represented in a glycaemic index and can be further rated according to the size of portion (giving the glycaemic load).

Vegetarian and vegan diets
Avoiding meat is not a problem as long as you get sufficient protein and iron from other sources, including pulses, beans, nuts, seeds and green vegetables. If you do not eat fish, eat linseeds regularly (1–2 tablespoons a day) or take a supplement, for omega oils. If you have a dairy-free diet, as long as it is carefully planned you can get enough nutrients: include nuts, seeds, pulses, cereals, leafy vegetables, beans and soya milk and tofu. (See also the vegetarian website www.vegsoc.org/info/preg.html.)

Supplementing safely
All women are advised to take folic acid supplements for protection against spina bifida and other neural tube defects. Other supplements will ensure you get the nutrients that you and your baby need. Since deficiencies in vitamins and minerals can contribute to a variety of problems,

Good for you

Vegetables and fruit
- ▶ Packed with vitamins and minerals, while fibre in the skins aids digestion
- ▶ Eat in abundance, raw, steamed, stir-fried or stewed

Potatoes, oats, wheat, bread, rice and pasta
- ▶ Complex carbohydrates with slow energy release
- ▶ Choose wholewheat/brown varieties, which have a nutty flavour and give energy for longer
- ▶ Cut back on pasta and bread if these make you feel bloated

Oily fish, e.g. sardines, mackerel, salmon, kippers, trout
- ▶ Contain protein and are an excellent source of essential fatty acids – aim for three portions/week
- ▶ Grill or bake to keep in the goodness

Meat, dairy products, lentils, pulses and beans
- ▶ All good sources of protein
- ▶ Eat red meat and dairy products in moderation
- ▶ Go easy on pulses and beans if they give you wind

Nuts, seeds and oils
- ▶ For general goodness but mostly for their essential fats (omega oils): these are essential for cell development, for you and for your baby, and for brain growth
- ▶ Omega oils are in linseeds (pre-cracked), hemp oil, walnut oil, oily fish, olive oil, sesame and sunflower oils

Food to avoid

Certain foods carry a high risk of infection that could affect your baby:
- ▶ Unpasteurised milk, cream and cheeses
- ▶ Blue-veined cheeses (e.g. Cambozola, Stilton) and soft cheeses (e.g. Brie, Camembert)
- ▶ Sheep cheese, which tends to be unpasteurised, as do some goats' cheeses
- ▶ Pâté and uncooked meats
- ▶ Raw fish and sushi
- ▶ Raw egg (including in dessert mousse, mayonnaise)
- ▶ Animal liver and fish liver oils, which have very high levels of vitamin A (in excess this may affect your baby's eye or brain development)

Buy organic whenever possible to avoid exposure to pesticides, hormones and antibiotics. You may need to take extra care if you have a health concern, such as diabetes or IBS.

must know

Take care
If you have an
allergy or a family
history of allergies,
take advice from a
qualified allergy
specialist while
you are pregnant
and in your baby's
early years.

ranging from fatigue and grumpiness to anaemia, it's wise to take the extra.

Choose a good-quality, general multivitamin and mineral designed for pregnancy. This will contain most of the basics, except for vitamin A, which is best avoided. The iron content may make your stools darker or harder. If constipation becomes a problem, consider changing your supplement.

Drinking for health

You need fluid, and the best way to get it is as still, unadulterated water. Aim for at least six glasses a day – easy to achieve if you have one when you wake or with breakfast; one mid-morning; one at lunch; two in the afternoon, and one with your evening meal.

For variety, you could squeeze fresh juices or make smoothies, and drink fruit and herb teas. Most benefit digestion. Keep Indian tea to a minimum (it stops your body from absorbing vitamins) and cut right down on coffee. If you have a heavy caffeine habit, reduce your intake gradually.

Alcohol

A little drop of wine or beer now and then – no more than one glass a week – probably has no ill effect. The opinions vary but it is wise to err on the side of caution and avoid alcohol. Drinking large amounts may impact your baby's development and could lead to foetal alcohol syndrome. This could manifest with, among other things, slow growth (IUGR), irritability and a tendency to addiction in later life.

Many women have a heavy night out before they are aware of pregnancy. Steer clear of alcohol as soon as you know you're pregnant and ask for monitoring if you're concerned. If you cannot kick an alcohol habit, seek support – you can do this in confidence (see website www.alcoholics-anonymous.org.uk).

Get shopping

Find out where your nearest organic or farmers' market is – these typically have a good variety of fresh foods and exquisite pickles, jams, pies, fresh juices and more. The prices often compare favourably with supermarket foods that are not so fresh, are higher in chemical residues and have clocked up many more miles in transit.

Get planting

You can bring delicious living food into your home – this is possible even in a flat, but if you have a garden, all the better. Try filling hanging baskets or pots with baby tomatoes and line your windowsills or doorstep with herbs. They taste great and have lots of health benefits: coriander is rich in iron; mint and dill aid digestion and reduce flatulence; thyme reduces abdominal cramps; parsley relieves swelling and is high in iron; and celery supports your kidneys. You could also sprout alfalfa seeds, which are rich in vitamin K and will help your blood to clot, reducing the risks of heavy bleeding after birth.

Basil adds excitement to tomato salads or soup, and is great with fish or pasta.

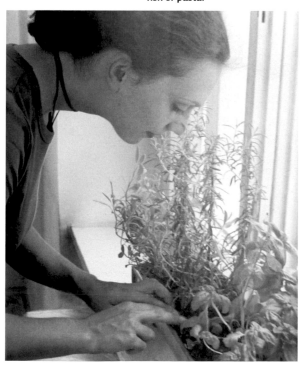

Weight in pregnancy

Weight gain in pregnancy is a cause for celebration: it's a good sign that your body is changing and your baby is growing. But how much is enough?

Step by step

Ideally, you'll gain gradually throughout pregnancy. Usually the greatest gain is in the second trimester (weeks 13–26), but this isn't universally true.

▶ Average gain in weeks 1–12: 1.4–1.8kg (3–4lb). Not gaining at all, or losing a little weight, is seldom a problem.

▶ In the second trimester, gain speeds up to 225–450g (1/2–1lb) per week.

▶ In the third trimester, the rate is similar. Weight gain may slow in the final month.

See box below for recommended overall weight gain.

Recommended overall weight gain

Starting BMI	Recommended overall gain
19.7 and below	12.7–18.2kg (28–40lb)
19.8–26	11.4–16kg (25–35¼lb)
27–29	6.8–9.1 kg (15–20lb)
30–40	not more than 6.8kg (15lb)
Twins	15.9–20.5kg (35–45lb)

Calculating your BMI

▶ Divide your weight in kg by your height in metres squared.

▶ So, a woman who weighs 60kg and is 1.6m (= 2.56m when squared) tall will have a BMI of 23.4. The recommended weight gain for her would be between 11.4 and 16kg (25 and 35¼lb).

What contributes?

Your baby accounts for only one quarter to a third of your overall gain. Additional weight comes from your fat stores, your own raised blood and fluid levels, your uterus, the amniotic fluid, the placenta and your enlarging breasts.

After birth, it may take 4–12 months to get back to your pre-pregnancy weight. Don't rush weight loss: try to focus on eating well, not on the scales.

Too much?

The most likely cause of excessive weight gain is too many calories. Remember: you're not eating for two adults. If you do, you may unwittingly contribute to excessive weight gain for your baby (see page 177) and this can increase the chance of difficulties in labour.

Women who gain heavily often review their diet and cut down on saturated fats, sugar and fruit juices. If you begin to gain more than 1kg (2lb) a week, particularly if you feel bloated and swollen, visit your midwife: this may be a sign of pre-eclampsia (page 169).

Too little?

If your weight gain is insufficient in the second or third trimester, your midwife may want to keep an eye on you. It's most likely that gain will pick up. Your team may check your baby's growth more frequently. If there is an identified cause (such as excessive vomitting, page 178), you will be given medical care and may receive fluid and nutrients via a drip.

Your feelings

You might excel in your new size and shape, but not everyone loves being bigger. This is truest in a first pregnancy: the sensation of carrying the extra weight can be strange. So if you are feeling low, try the tips in the box above right.

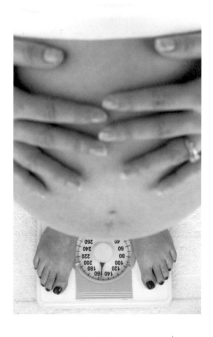

Exercise and relax

Exercising and relaxing are essential cogs in the wheel of life: without them, body, mind and spirit fall out of balance. With them, your physical health and emotional wellbeing will improve, and you'll also be preparing yourself for labour, birth and beyond.

watch out!

Feeling breathless or faint?
If you feel breathless, faint or dizzy, stop exercising immediately. If you experience pain or bleeding, you need to tell your midwife or doctor straight away.

Exercise for love and comfort

Exercise is good for you – it tones and strengthens your muscles and bones and it sends feel-good and love hormones through your body and to your baby. It also assists digestion and can help to relieve food cravings. But there's no need to go crazy in pregnancy; in fact, quite the opposite. You need to listen to your body and avoid becoming over-heated or tired. If you cannot talk during exercise, you are working yourself too hard.

Unless there's a physical problem that is preventing you from getting out and about, aim to exercise for 20–30 minutes a day, or at least every other day. Combine this with balanced meals and drink plenty of water before, during and after exercise. Ask your midwife or doctor to confirm that what you're doing is safe at each stage in pregnancy. If you plan to do any exercise you haven't done before, take advice.

In the first trimester you need to be gentle. Don't do anything you are not already used to, and cut down rather than build up your regime. Regular walking may be best, and it's fine to do some every day. Avoid high intensity aerobics or running and twists and seek advice for any exercise – even pilates or yoga – from a qualified teacher. The general advice is to hold back until after the first trimester.

Aerobic and anaerobic exercise
During aerobic exercise the aim is to raise your heartbeat slightly without becoming breathless. Walking is perfect and will get you

out into the fresh air. Swimming is also excellent and extremely relaxing, but avoid breaststroke if you have pelvic pain. You can join antenatal swimming or aqua yoga groups from week 20.

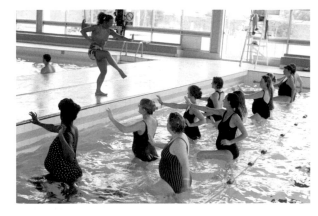

Anaerobic exercise focuses on stretching with easy breath. Exercises work with the natural softening of your body's muscles and ligaments to enhance your posture and flexibility and help you to tone your abdominal and pelvic muscles. Antenatal exercise classes are suitable after week 24; yoga or pilates are suitable from week 13. Always stretch comfortably: don't take any joint to its maximum.

Antenatal stretches

A gentle sequence of these antenatal exercises could be part of your regular yoga routine (see page 30) or may be new to you. Find a class and/or a good book to guide you through exercises that focus on your pelvis, abdominal muscles, shoulders, neck, thighs and calves.

If you choose swimming (which may range from aqua-aerobics to aqua-yoga), the water holds your weight and encourages the flow of relaxing and pain-relieving hormones.

After birth

Ease yourself back into exercise gently. You can begin pelvic tilts and tightenings within days; and gentle yoga within five to ten days. Begin aerobic exercise with short walks and build up gradually. Your body takes time to return to pre-pregnancy tone and strength. If you have a caesarean section, avoid aerobic exercise apart from walking for ten weeks.

For more information, see *The Body Control Pilates Pregnancy Book* by Lynne Robinson and *Aqua Yoga for Pregnancy* by Françoise Barbira Freeman.

Chilling out

Relaxing may involve anything from watching a movie to enjoying a meal out or meditating. Spending time in water, listening to music or doing yoga may do it for you. If you enjoy a massage, try lemon oil to boost your energy; neroli to promote sleep; and try ylang ylang or sandalwood if you are afraid or depressed.

You can also look to your baby for peace. Place your hands on your abdomen and tune in. You might want to tell her about your feelings or some gifts you'd like to give her – strength, beauty, wit, joy, humour – you can do this alone and with your partner.

As you relax, remember your posture, so that you and your baby are comfortable. Sit with your back supported so that your breathing is easy and you're not slouching. Good posture may also benefit your baby (see page 100).

Drugs

If you use drugs to relax or to stay awake, your baby will experience the same highs and lows as you do, and her brain development can be affected. Potentially harmful substances include alcohol, amphetamines, cocaine, ecstasy, LSD, nicotine, marijuana, opium, crack, smack, heroin and some medicines. Continued use and high doses pose the greatest hazard.

You may be nervous if you have taken one or more drugs. You can ask for ultrasound scans to check your baby. If you're stuck, do seek help. Complementary therapies such as acupuncture may help you break the habit. Talk to your doctor or midwife; they can help and need to know if your personal history could be relevant during labour. If you're a smoker, try Allen Carr's book *How to Stop Smoking*. A counsellor may help you resolve some of the underlying issues that fuel your habit.

Yoga

Yoga is one of the best labour preparations for your mind and body and it's a great way to keep you chilled and comfortable through pregnancy. You don't have to be a professional: whether you have been practising for years or begin in pregnancy, it has immense benefits.

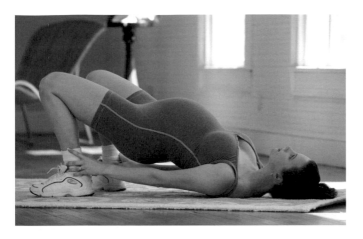

good to know

Health
► Until week 13, focus on seated exercises and breathing.
► If you have any health problems or complications with pregnancy, check with your doctor that yoga is safe for you and ask your teacher for advice.
► If any position feels uncomfortable, stop: yoga is meant to be pleasurable, it is not a competition.

Yoga postures combine gentle effort and relaxation, awareness of breath and concentration on body and mind. The exercise stretches and massages your body, inside and out, to reduce aches and pains and boost your immunity and sense of wellbeing.

For many women, the best thing about yoga is the freedom it brings from anxieties and schedules. Quiet time will help you become aware of what you and your baby need and to follow your instincts. You may combine your yoga with meditation. The simplest meditation is to focus on your breath, on a short 'mantra' or set of words or on an image. This trains your mind to be in the 'here and now', undistracted by thoughts about the future and the past. Scientific research into meditation (even the Dalai Lama has been hooked up to neuroscience monitors) shows many benefits, including stabilization of blood pressure and circulation, unrestricted flow of hormones and profound relaxation.

To find out more, try www.bwy.org.uk, or, for contacts in your area, look at local noticeboards. Other websites include www.birthlight.com and www.activebirthcentre.com/pb/catyogaforpregnancy. See also *Yoga for Pregnancy* by Françoise Barbira Freedman.

Work: your entitlements

If you are working, you may need to adapt while you are pregnant and will certainly need to plan for time off. The first step is to consider your entitlements. You may also want to think about flexible hours, job sharing, or even taking a long-term break once your baby is born.

Sit down for your rights

Sitting down all day won't do you any favours while you're pregnant, and nor will being on your feet all day long. While you're at work, eat well, aim for a balance of rest and activity and remember you are entitled to request a change in role or removal from a hazardous situation.

Maternity leave

You are entitled to 26 weeks maternity leave as long as you have been in your job for at least 26 weeks prior to week 25 before your baby is due.

▶ You may start your leave at any time from the beginning of week 29.
▶ You are legally required to inform your employer by week 25.

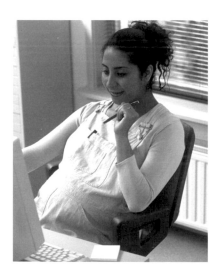

Statutory maternity pay (SMP)

You qualify for 26 weeks' SMP if your employer contributes Class 1 National Insurance payments on your behalf. For the first six weeks of absence you are entitled to 90% of your average earnings. For the remaining 20 weeks, you are entitled to a certain amount each week or 90% of your average earnings, whichever is lower. You may be offered a different depending on your circumstances.

If you're sitting a lot, walk and stretch every 40 minutes to loosen your body and your mind.

Maternity Allowance

You may claim Maternity Allowance from Jobcentre Plus if you do not qualify for SMP, for instance if your earnings are low, you have not been working in your current job for long enough, or you are self-employed. You must have been working in at least 26 weeks out of the 66 weeks prior to your due date. If so, you qualify for a certain amount each week for 26 weeks or 90% of your average earnings, whichever is lower. You can find out more from your nearest job centre or social security office.

good to know

Flexible working
Every parent is entitled to ask for flexible working hours and by law the request must be considered. You're also entitled to take up to 13 weeks unpaid leave to care for your child, should she need it, within five years of her birth.

Additional maternity leave

It's now legal to request up to 26 weeks leave in addition to the first period of 26 weeks maternity leave. The extra is, typically, unpaid.

Paternity leave

The year 2005 finally saw the introduction of paternity leave. Although short, at one to two weeks, it's a positive start. The qualifications for leave and the levels of payment are the same as for women, but the period to which you are entitled is just two weeks. You must take one or two weeks consecutive leave – you cannot cherry pick days here and there.

To make the most of your paternity leave, it may be best not to overlap with other helpers such as your mother-in-law or a maternity nurse. You might want to consider extending your leave with holiday entitlement.

Standing up for your rights

Getting maternity or paternity leave and payment is a right that's seldom refused. Unfortunately, while some work places are parent-friendly and even exceptionally considerate, some can be unsympathetic. If you feel you are being pressurized or bullied, do seek support. Begin with the Citizens Advice Bureau (CAB; www.cab.co.uk) or your company's complaints office. Sticking up for your rights is exhausting – make sure you have friends around you.

Sex

Sex in pregnancy is not often talked about, but it is a shame: it's incredibly important. Almost all couples experience change. Sex might be brilliant, perhaps with multiple orgasms for the first time, or it may not feature for you. There is no right or wrong, feelings change from day to day and both partners don't always feel the same.

good to know

Enjoying sex

▶ Female orgasm is good for you. It relaxes you, your uterus pulses with contractions that massage your baby, and your body is flooded with hormones that make you and your baby feel high. Enjoying orgasm may be a great release from anxiety.

▶ Getting into satisfying positions, particularly in the last trimester, can be challenging. Seated postures, penetration from behind and 'spooning' can work well and there's even more variation with oral sex.

Intimacy

Good sex, or closeness without sexual contact, is based on emotional and physical intimacy. You may want to deepen this aspect of your relationship during quiet moments together. Exploring one another's bodies, perhaps sharing a bath or massage might be fun.

It's often easier to maintain intimacy after birth if you develop your menu during pregnancy. If intimacy is lacking or feels wrong, the best starting point is to talk: aim for a time when you can be together without distractions.

He wants sex but I don't

Most men have powerful sex drives and need an outlet for this. You could encourage your partner to get into his natural energy and if you enjoy massages, for instance, he may get pleasure from this. If you don't enjoy his touch, he may expend energy with vigorous exercise and self-pleasure. If you feel guilty, remember that your libido is heavily influenced by your pregnancy and you will feel sexy again in the future.

You can still enjoy your sensuality by dressing beautifully (including stunning underwear) and stroking your body with luxurious body oil; and enjoy intimacy without sexual contact.

For some women, sexual contact is a catalyst for fears around sex and birth to surface. If this happens, do talk about it. Working through your fears will help you feel more confident in labour and birth.

I want sex but he doesn't

When men go off sex it's usually because they don't want to be close to the baby or do not fancy their partners. If this is your experience, you can use the chance to seduce and pleasure yourself – it's a great opportunity to indulge and to learn and perhaps to feel more closely in touch with your vagina in advance of birth. Letting your sexual energy flow may set you up well for birth when self-expression can help progress.

After the birth

The big question – when will we do it again? – has a different answer for each couple. You may have sex again within two weeks or not for ten or more months. Much depends on how each of you reacts to the birth, postnatal recovery, whether you are tired, and how much time you have together.

For women, the most common anxiety is that sex will be painful. Take it easy. Using KY jelly or a natural oil may help and it may be easiest with the woman on top. Your vagina may feel and appear different following birth but it may still feel tight, with control improving as your pregnancy hormones dissipate and your tissues heal (keep up pelvic floor exercises).

If you have pain, do tell your doctor at your six-week check or book an appointment for a gynaecology check. Some women find birth traumatic or feel their vagina and privacy have been violated. Consider visiting an experienced counsellor who can help you get back in touch with a fulfilling part of you.

must know

Sex and safety
Sexual arousal, orgasm, oral sex and penetrative sex are completely safe throughout pregnancy *unless* you experience bleeding. If you have a history of miscarriage, abstain from penetration until week 13. If your waters break, abstain from sexual intercourse to avoid the risk of introducing bacteria into your womb.

Planning ahead

Planning ahead for what lies beyond birth can be part of the fun of pregnancy. The most basic needs for your family and your baby are love, warmth, food and shelter: the more elaborate could include electronic temperature monitors, multi-tasking baby-seats, musical mobiles and more. So where do you strike the balance?

Bare essentials

If you have a tendency to buy and collect more than you need or have no idea what's essential, use the suggestions below as a guide.

For your baby: clothes

▶ 6 vests
▶ 6 babygros, front opening with poppers
▶ 3 cardigans
▶ 5 pairs socks or booties
▶ Scratch mitts (only use if your baby scratches – otherwise let her suck her fingers and use them to explore)
▶ 10 bibs
▶ 2 hats – one thin, one thick (remember that your baby will lose heat from her head)
▶ 1 coat
▶ In winter, 1 warm all-in-one suit to wear outdoors.

For your baby: equipment

▶ Nappies: check web and magazine listings for biodegradable disposables and washable varieties. Initially buy 40 newborn disposable nappies or 10 washable ones and see how you get on. Test for absorbability and ease of use. For tips, try www.realnappycampaign.com and www.wen.org.uk.

▶ Moses basket with new mattress. You may prefer a cot that slots onto the side of your bed.

▶ Cot and new mattress (although the Moses basket may be sufficient for three or more months).

▶ Well-fitting sheets and cellular blankets: always choose natural fabrics (cotton/wool).

▶ Baby wipes, unscented.

▶ 2 changing mats (one for the home and a roll-up one for going out).

▶ Things for your baby to look at (see page 155).

▶ Car seat: safety is paramount. You may need to spend some time choosing the seat that's right for your car. Newer models recline fully to give the best possible support.

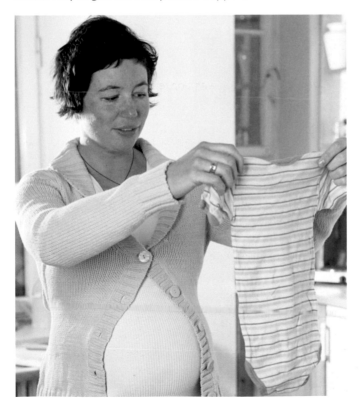

Pack a few babygros with nappies and your personal clothes in a bag for hospital.

▶ Pram or a pushchair that fully reclines. Pushchairs with raised backs are no use until four to six months.

▶ Plastic baby bath (although using the adult bath with mum or dad is lovely for a baby).

▶ Soft cotton wool: use with water to wash her.

▶ Pure olive oil, almond oil or grapeseed oil for massaging and protecting her skin.

Day to day

▶ Muslin squares – invaluable for catching milk and sick.

▶ Bottle-feeding kit (if you plan to bottle feed), including sterilizer.

▶ Baby monitor to use if your baby is sleeping somewhere out of your ear shot.

▶ Comfortable backpack that will contain all your kit while you're out.

▶ Breast pump: don't express to feed until eight weeks, but expressing may relieve discomfort in the early days (page 158).

For you after birth

▶ Breast pads: washable cloth or disposable.

▶ Maternity/heavy-flow sanitary towels.

▶ Postnatal bath soak, made from natural ingredients.

▶ Dressing gown or 'easy' clothes for relaxing at home, with breast access.

For you and your partner

▶ Supportive sling: choose something that fits both parents and allows your baby to snuggle into your chest and, from eight to ten weeks, to face out to the world. Being carried is the next best thing to being in the womb and it helps to strengthen your baby's muscles and spine. For you, the carrying helps your bones build strength and protects against osteoporosis.

Optional extras

▶ Baby gym: some babies seem to enjoy lying under a baby gym very early on; others don't get much out of them until five, six or seven weeks ….

▶ Breastfeeding pillow: a padded 'V' shape can take strain off your shoulders and help your baby stay comfortable. It doubles up as a prop when your baby starts sitting and tumbling.

▶ Baby sleeping bag.

Cleaning products

There's a vast market devoted to toiletries for babies. It's ironic because a baby doesn't need any heavily processed chemicals. Your baby's skin protects and cleanses itself, if it isn't hindered. Chemical products can stop skin from breathing and reduce its capacity to moisturize and clean itself. And because skin is highly absorbent, the whole body is affected by what goes onto the skin.

Look after your baby's skin by washing her gently with lukewarm water and drying with a soft towel. Use 100% natural products to nurture rather than drain her skin. Massage with oil, such as olive, grapeseed or almond, or use a pure baby oil that's infused with essential oils like lavender. Oil around her nappy area will be soothing and protective. Test every product on a 1cm (1/2in)-square patch of your baby's skin for a reaction over a 24-hour period.

People power

Planning ahead includes planning extra help – in the run up to labour, while you're in hospital and for days, weeks or months afterwards. Parents, sisters, relatives, friends, or nanny or maternity nurse: whatever suits you. Doulas are becoming more widely used: women who are themselves mothers and help out prenatally, at birth, and/or afterwards (see page 46). Knowing you have a support network can greatly reduce anxiety about coping after birth. Remember that support does not only focus on your baby: any relief from day-to-day chores will help you relax and enjoy the early days.

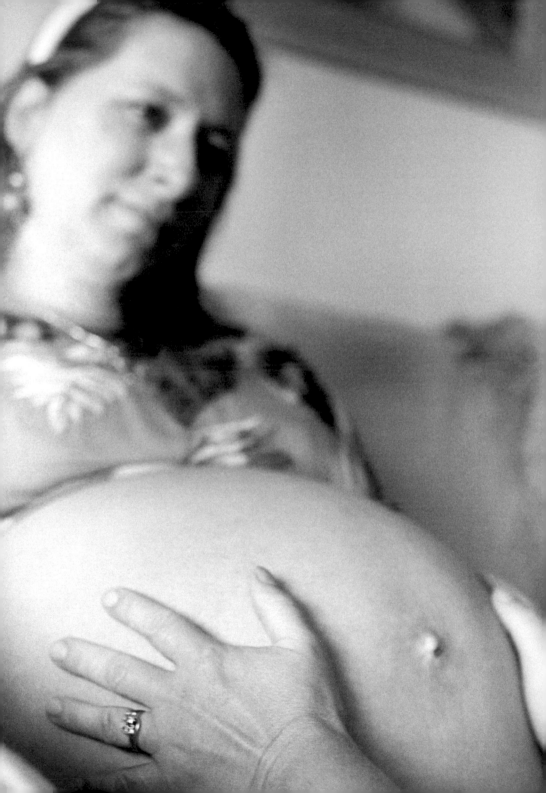

2 Healthcare

Pregnancy is not a medical condition, nor is labour an emergency. But because both may potentially involve health concerns it is important to be closely cared for. Antenatal testing is part of this. The midwives and other specialists you meet are not simply monitoring you: they may also protect and empower you on your journey, and will be there for you if any problems arise. Feeling loved, informed and encouraged is known to enhance birth satisfaction and postnatal recovery.

'... in all fields of medicine, there have been studies revealing correlations between an adult disease and what happened when the mother was pregnant. It is even possible to conclude that our health is to a great extent shaped in the womb. There are in particular many studies confirming the emotional states of pregnant women may have life-long effects on their children. This leads to the conclusion that the first duty of health professionals should be to deal tactfully with the emotional state of pregnant women.'
Michel Odent, from *Birth and Breastfeeding*

Medical care

Your medical support may be rooted in midwifery care, or it may extend to include several specialists. Close medical care, with antenatal visits and monitoring, ensures that your safety is always prioritised, and gives regular opportunities for you to ask questions, discuss your feelings and learn more about your baby.

Your GP

Your GP will probably be the first medical professional you see. She will explain your local antenatal care system and answer your questions. You may not see her again until your six-week check after birth; although it's a good idea to pay her one or two visits. After birth she will be the main carer for your family. A small number of GPs also deliver babies (see page 58).

Your midwives

Midwives are the guardians of birth and are at the heart of antenatal and birth care. Midwifery is an art. A good midwife can often tell how a woman feels by her mood and appearance, and whether there may be problems. Experienced midwives combine this special wisdom with modern medical skills and some also practise complementary skills such as aromatherapy and massage (pages 46 and 47). In pregnancy, you can talk to your midwife about tests and your hopes for labour and birth. During labour, one or more midwives will help you through your journey. After birth, midwives check your baby and help you establish feeding and hold and care for your baby. They also care for you and support you if you are not feeling good. You will be visited at home by a midwife for up to 14 days after birth.

must know

Midwife meetings
1 Around week 6–10: booking visit on confirmation of pregnancy.
2 Until week 32: one visit every month, more frequently if you need extra care.
3 Beyond week 32: one to two visits every month.
4 Beyond week 36: one visit each week.

You will meet one or more community midwives at intervals through pregnancy. If you wish to give birth in hospital, you may have a chance to meet the midwife team there. It is also possible to hire an independent midwife (see www.maternallink.com).

Your obstetrician

An obstetrician is a doctor trained in caring for women during childbirth and in pregnancy. On the NHS all women are appointed a consultant obstetrician to oversee their care and have a chance to meet their consultant at least once in pregnancy; sometimes more frequently. Your care may be consultant-led, which means you may see your obstetrician as regularly as you see your midwife if you have special medical needs. You may request consultant-led care if you go private.

Your appointed consultant may be working at the time you go into labour, and if you need an obstetric opinion or extra care, she will be called. It is equally likely, though, that another obstetrician will be on duty. You may have a chance to meet the team prior to labour.

Your paediatrician

A paediatrician is a doctor trained to care for babies and children. All babies are checked by a paediatrician within 72 hours of birth. If antenatal monitoring has raised concerns, your paediatrician may talk to you about the specific issue, and advise you on the timing and manner of birth. She will also be present to check your baby at birth. If your baby needs special care, your paediatrician may become an important member of your support team for weeks, months or years to come.

Other medical carers

Other people you may meet include ultrasound specialists in pregnancy and any specialists you need (e.g. diabetic care team). You may meet an anaesthetist if you choose to have epidural pain relief during labour, or if you require a caesarean.

Complementary therapies

Integrated healthcare – where conventional medical care is used alongside complementary therapies – is becoming increasingly popular in the UK. It is particularly suitable in pregnancy, when unpleasant symptoms are common yet many medical procedures and drugs are off-limits.

Why choose complementary therapies?

Complementary care works with your mind and body in unison: treatments aim to improve both your mental and physical wellbeing and may have a spiritual element too. You may use complementary therapies to address a concerning issue; but they are also valuable to boost general health, to help you avoid preventable problems, to help you prepare for labour and to aid your recovery after birth.

Many professionals claim that a woman's vital energy becomes stronger in pregnancy, when the influences of gentle therapies can be especially effective.

You may be able to use complementary care during labour: given either by a trained therapist or by your birth partner, if adequately trained. If you wish to have a professional with you in hospital, you will need to arrange this with the maternity unit; at home you will need to discuss it with your community midwife.

watch out!

Medical conditions
If you have any known or suspected medical condition, tell your therapist. You also need to tell your midwife and doctor if you are receiving complementary care.

Which therapy for you?

The range of complementary therapies available is vast. We cover just a few here (see overleaf). Before you go ahead, check out the therapist's credentials and experience in caring for women in pregnancy. The way you and the therapist get along is vitally important: if you feel comfortable and confident this will enhance the effect of treatment. Side effects with the therapies listed are extremely uncommon. If you choose to use herbs, which can be highly potent, you must seek specialist advice.

Complementary therapies and their benefits

Here is a quick guide to a few of the options that might help you. In some hospitals and health centres, certain complementary therapies are available to all women who request them. It is more common, though, for families to find their own complementary practitioners.

Acupuncture

This element of traditional Chinese medicine has been in use for over 2000 years. Acupuncture uses needles to stimulate and balance energy. It impacts emotions, muscle tension, hormone balance, and can be used to support a healthy uterine environment and a baby's optimal growth. It's particularly good for nausea and morning sickness; stress relief; back pain in pregnancy; addressing addictions; pain relief in labour. With herbal remedies (moxibustion), acupuncture has very high rates of success turning breech babies. **Good to know** that if you do not like needles, the principles of acupuncture can be applied with acupressure (finger pressure/massage).

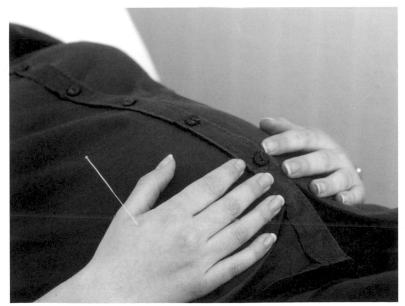

For induction, an acupuncture needle in the 'colon four' point, with others, helps to descend the baby. It's a 'no-go' point at any other time of pregnancy.

Aromatherapy

An ancient tradition drawing on herbal wisdom, aromatherapy uses essential oils from plants during massage, for inhalation and in water for bathing. It taps into your sense of smell and the healing properties are absorbed by your skin. It's good for relaxation and pain relief; to reduce headaches and nausea; and to relieve stress; easy to use in labour provided you are informed about safety. **Good to know** that you must take guidance; some oils, such as lavender, need to be avoided in early pregnancy; and there are some that must be avoided at all times.

Counselling/psychotherapy

Counselling is an age-old tradition, but psychotherapy evolved in the 20th century. These provide space and guidance for you to express what's on your mind and explore difficult feelings or focus on challenging situations. It's particularly good for relieving stress, improving your confidence and self-esteem and working through relationship problems. Most people who are depressed or have experienced loss or trauma find emotional therapy extremely helpful. **Good to know** that in pregnancy women and men alike can become emotionally sensitive and difficult issues arise – pregnancy may be an opportunity to clear the cobwebs in readiness for parenthood.

Doulas

Meaning 'handmaidens', doulas are becoming increasingly popular, offering one-to-one support during birth and/or postnatally. The emphasis is on personal and loving care; the doula does not play the medical role of a midwife. Most doulas are mothers whose presence may make a potentially anxious experience enjoyable, and their presence reduces the chance of complications. After birth, doulas help mums and dads to settle into parenting. **Good to know** that doulas need to be hired privately. Many are also trained in aromatherapy, massage, etc. See www.doula.org.uk.

Homeopathy

Homeopathy has been in use for over 200 years. It uses the principle of 'like cures like'; remedies trigger a healing response to restore physical and emotional balance. It's great for all antenatal and postnatal ailments and an excellent support for labour (for men too). Homeopathy works well in conjunction with medical care to reduce potential side effects. **Good to know** that it can be used for babies from birth; aids postnatal healing; and offers support for breastfeeding.

Massage

This instinctive therapy, as old as childbirth itself, uses pressure to relieve tension and pain and rebalance your energy. A practitioner may also draw on reflexology, focusing on the soles of your feet. The effects include pain relief, hormone balance, improved organ function, and flexibility. It's particularly good for relaxation and pain relief; improving sleep; preparing your vagina and perineum to stretch at birth. If you enjoy practising at home, massage may enhance intimacy in your partnership. **Good to know** that baby massage has immense and life long benefits (page 155).

Osteopathy

Founded in 1874, osteopathy supports your bones, muscles, ligaments, organs, nerves and fluid systems. Cranial osteopathy is the most gentle and is preferred in pregnancy and for treating babies. It's good for pain relief, especially in your back, head, neck and pelvis. For you and your baby, it helps to relieve nerve, skeletal, muscular and emotional tension that can arise from compression, pressure or trauma in pregnancy or during birth, especially when there has been intervention. **Good to know** that you may be referred for osteopathic treatment in the NHS.

Visualization

An ancient and widespread practice, visualization relaxes and helps you work towards your goals; many people believe that regular visualizations can influence reality. Guided visualizations are very powerful and may involve some hypnotherapy or self-hypnosis. You may use it to relieve anxiety and to encourage your cervix to ripen and your baby and pelvis to prepare for birth (see page 91). Visualization comes into its own in labour, when it may reduce stress and boost progress. **Good to know** that you can still use visualizations for relaxation when you breastfeed and at other times after birth.

Antenatal classes and groups

Almost all pregnant women and, increasingly commonly, expectant dads go to at least one antenatal class in the run up to labour. These are for you to find out what you can expect, to meet others in a similar situation, and to prepare your body and mind for labour and for parenting. Many antenatal groups hold postnatal reunions.

must know
Natural birth
Some women feel pressurized to 'achieve' natural birth as the ultimate goal and to follow all the advice given. Please take advice but remember that your own experience will be unique; use what you learn as a tool rather than as a standard you need to live up to.

Community groups

Community midwives run regular groups for women at any stage after week 28 in hospital or in a local health centre or village hall. They are free of charge and are often attended only by women, although there may be couples classes as well. The midwife will guide you through topics including normal labour and birth, pain relief, intervention and breast- and bottle feeding – and there is always time for tea and a chat. Use the space to share your stories and ask questions; for instance, if you want to know more about caesarean section, delivering your placenta or breech birth.

The National Childbirth Trust (NCT) groups are extremely popular. A course runs for two hours a week over eight weeks, and may be in the evening: you are encouraged to attend as a couple. The NCT encourages informed choice and active birth: there will be practice of positions and perhaps breathing techniques. The groups are informal and many continue with postnatal and toddler meetings. Each group has its own website: for general information and prices, go to www.nctpregnancyandbabycare.com.

Antenatal exercise classes

Run by qualified teachers, these provide the perfect opportunity to ease aches and pains, relax and prepare your body for birth. Check out classified sections in magazines, noticeboards and the web, and see page 30 for yoga information.

Antenatal testing and screening

Being screened through pregnancy is one of today's health choices. This means we can choose to know more about our babies than ever before, and there may be options for beneficial care if something is amiss. Knowing what the tests entail will help you make your own choices.

Routine monitoring

Tests carried out at each antenatal visit monitor your wellbeing and screen for signs that you are unwell and, later in pregnancy, that you may be at risk of complications in labour. At each visit (see page 42), your midwife will ask to check a combination of factors: your blood pressure, weight, urine, the feel of your abdomen and your baby's heartbeat.

Standard tests

During pregnancy, a number of tests are available to you – they may be presented as standard, yet all are optional. They typically include ultrasound scans and blood tests, used as a primary means of assessing whether anything about you, your baby or your pregnancy deviates from the norm.

To know or not to know?

Tests usually give reassuring results and a sense of security; and with ultrasound, seeing your baby may be a wonderful and very moving experience. They also help to prevent potential problems (e.g. if an infection can be tackled). Yet with tests that can reveal – or raise a suspicion of – developmental problems, the information may trigger anxiety and could lead to stressful choices. Before you have developmental checks you may want to consider. What is the accuracy? Are there risks? How much do you want to know? Would you consider a termination? Do you want to know as much as possible as you prepare for life beyond birth? These questions are difficult but important, and it is worth exploring them with your partner and/or a close friend or advisor.

Antenatal tests

Screening for congenital abnormalities is central to antenatal care. Tests for Down's syndrome and neural tube defects are now offered to most women in the UK. There is an important distinction between screening tests and diagnostic tests:

▶ A screening test gives an indication of risk.

▶ A diagnostic test gives a definite diagnosis.

You only need to consider having a diagnostic test if your personal risk factor is high.

Screening tests

Nuchal translucency (NT) scan

Date	Checks for	Time for results
Weeks 10–14	Down's syndrome markers	At the time of scanning

Accuracy In the hands of an experienced operator, the scan detects 60% of babies who are affected. It has a false positive rate of 5% (see page 53)

First trimester maternal serum screen (FTMSS) blood test

Date	Checks	Time for results
Weeks 10–14	Your blood group, rhesus factor, and signs of viral infection (e.g. syphilis, HIV, rubella)	Up to 2 weeks

Accuracy Blood group and rhesus factor are clear. You may be re-tested to confirm a suspected antibody presence

Alphafetoprotein (AFP) blood test

Date	Checks for	Time for results
Week 10–14	Looks for markers of genetic abnormalities in your baby	Up to 2 weeks

Accuracy Markers indicate risk and are considered together with ultrasound findings and your age and personal history to assess risk

Mouth wash and further blood tests

Date	Checks for	Time for results
Weeks 8–18	Cystic fibrosis (mouth wash); anaemia; hepatitis; Strep B	Various

Accuracy Detection of infection in adults is accurate. To ascertain the risk of your baby being affected, further tests may be offered.

Screening tests/cont.

'Triple' or 'double' blood test (or the second trimester maternal serum screen) (STMSS)

Date	Checks for	Time for results
Weeks 15–18	Spinal tube defects such as spina bifida and anencephaly; markers for Down's syndrome	Up to one week

Accuracy Around one in 20 women receive a 'screen positive' result indicating a raised risk; of these women around one in 50 has an affected baby. Your results will be used in conjunction with the NT scan and FTMSS results to estimate your overall risk

Second trimester ultrasound scan

Date	Purpose	Time for results
Weeks 16–20	Checks the internal structure of your baby e.g. brain, intestines diaphragm, heart and limbs	At the time of scanning

Accuracy Although scans do not pick up all abnormalities, accuracy is increasing. It is not possible, however, to predict the exact outcome of any structural abnormality

Integrated testing The most accurate screening results come from a combination of FTMSS and NT ultrasound scan at ten weeks as well as the second trimester blood test around week 16. Availability of this 'integrated testing' is promised on the NHS by 2007 and should reduce unnecessary amniocentesis procedures: it detects 90% of Down's syndrome babies and has a relatively low false positive rate of 3%.

Diagnostic tests

Chorionic villus sampling (cvs) (involves inserting a needle into the placenta via your abdomen or vagina)

Date	Purpose	Time for results
Weeks 11–12	Obtains cells from the placenta to analyze your baby's genes	2–14 days

Accuracy and risk Gives a good analysis of your baby's genes, but cannot test for every genetic problem. Carries a miscarriage risk ranging from 1:100 to 1:25

Amniocentesis (involves inserting a needle into the amniotic fluid via your abdomen)

Date	Purpose	Time for results
Weeks 15 16	Obtains cells from the amniotic fluid to check for spina bifida and genetic abnormalities	2–14 days

Accuracy and risk Gives a DNA profile but cannot test for every genetic problem. Carries a risk of miscarriage ranging from 1:50 to 1:200. It may also increase the risk of premature birth and low birth weight due to further interventions

Your age
The risk of a developmental
abnormality rises as your age
rises. This will be taken into
consideration when your risk is
estimated on the results of your
NT scan and your baby's
measurements in the first
trimester.

**With ultrasound, you can see
your baby while the specialist
observes the finer details.**

What does a positive screening test result mean?

If a screening test reveals you have a viral infection
or antibody deficiency, you may need treatment to
protect you and your baby.

Rhesus factor

Most people are rhesus positive, which means their
blood cells contain the rhesus factor, or a certain
protein. If, like 15% of people, you lack this protein
and are rhesus negative, there's no risk to you. Yet if
your baby is rhesus positive and your bloods mix,
either in pregnancy or during birth, your body could
react by producing antibodies. In a future pregnancy,
this could threaten a rhesus positive baby. If you are
rhesus negative, you will be offered an 'anti-D'
injection in pregnancy and again after birth; this

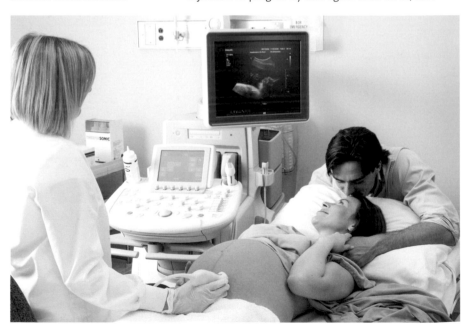

reduces the potential risks of miscarrying a rhesus positive baby in a future pregnancy.

Down's syndrome

Down's syndrome (see page 173) is a rare condition, yet it is the most common chromosomal abnormality. Many people with Down's syndrome have a good quality of life but there are challenges for them and their families. Some expectant parents wish to know whether their baby is affected because they either want to plan ahead for the future or because they would prefer to end the pregnancy if their baby is affected.

If your risk is high (usually more than 1:250), an amniocentesis or cvs is offered. You will be guided through this procedure by your midwife, doctor or genetic counsellor.

False positives, false negatives

Tests are offering increasingly accurate results yet there is still a margin of uncertainty and false positives do occur; that is, some women are given a high risk factor when there is no problem. If a test has a false positive result of 5%, for instance, this means that five in every 100 babies (that's one in every 20) said to be at risk are actually unaffected. False negatives also occur, when an abnormality goes undetected – as many as one in three babies with Down's syndrome are not detected through routine screening tests. Some conditions, such as cerebral palsy, autism and the majority of heart conditions, cannot be detected during pregnancy.

For more information, see www.arc-uk.org.

good to know

The safety of scanning
Ultrasound scanning has been in use for three decades. As yet there is no indication that it carries significant risks; at the same time, there is no definitive proof that it is entirely risk free.

Special care

As more is being understood about women and babies in pregnancy, treatments and precautionary measures are improving. In the vast majority of cases, a high-risk pregnancy continues without serious problems and babies who were considered to be at risk thrive after birth. Extra care is designed to minimize potential problems.

What is a high-risk pregnancy?

Despite the small number of women at increased risk, there are many conditions that are linked with potential complications in pregnancy or birth; most are covered briefly in the A–Z section (see pages 166–86).

Maternal issues that may complicate pregnancy range from diabetes and high blood pressure to obesity and infection. Concern may centre on a baby for reasons including intra-uterine growth restriction (IUGR), twins (or more), and, much less commonly, genetic abnormalities.

Your personal risk and the extent of care you will be offered depend on your circumstances, what has happened in any previous pregnancies, the history of medical problems in your family and your partner's family, and the indications of antenatal monitoring and test results. For some conditions, medical support is important, e.g. antibiotics to address infection, regular insulin for Type 1 diabetes, or medication for a chronic condition.

Monitoring

Increased monitoring may include blood, urine and other tests for you, as well as ultrasound scanning to check your baby and the function of your placenta. This ensures that, should a mild condition become severe or a complication arise, it will be detected as early as possible.

Emotional support

If you are told there is an increased risk for you or for your baby, you will understandably be anxious. Feeling heard and supported by your midwife

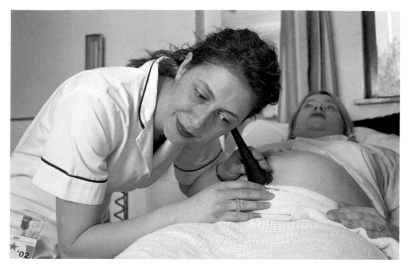

Foetal heart rate is a good measure of your baby's wellbeing.

and other members of your care team, will help. Further support at home, particularly within your partnership, will also be invaluable.

High-risk pregnancies are usually classified according to physical markers, yet maternal anxiety may contribute to premature birth, IUGR and slow progress and distress in labour. It may also contribute to postnatal depression. If you are at all anxious, practical help and having people to talk to could make a huge difference. If your anxiety is fuelled by medical concerns, your most helpful supporters may be midwives and professional counsellors.

Labour and birth

If you have a high-risk pregnancy, this will be noted by your birth team who will be alert for signs of distress in your baby during labour. You may need to give birth in a hospital where there are facilities for epidural and caesarean section and a special care baby unit.

After birth, your team may want to keep a close eye on you and/or your baby. What they are looking for depends on your personal issues. Your baby may need to be cared for by an experienced paediatrician. If the risk factors are significant, your baby may be offered tests, medication or treatment. The precise nature of care depends on your situation and you do have a say in your baby's care (see page 182).

Where do you want to give birth?

The birth environment – how safe you feel, what you see, what you smell, feel and hear, and who is with you – profoundly affects your emotions, the balance of hormones in your body and your sensitivity to pain. These play a central role in the way labour unfolds and how you and your baby experience birth.

Safe and sound

As recently as 40 years ago, most babies were born in their parents' home. In the UK today, only around one in 50 are born at home. This figure reflects a trend towards hospital care and the medicalization of labour; but there is no evidence of any difference in safety between home births and hospital births. The strongest evidence regarding labour is that the more relaxed, safe and comfortable a woman feels, the less likely it is that complications will arise.

Every woman is unique, and for you, feeling safe may mean being in a hospital; or it may mean being at home with familiar things around you. Your decision will also depend on where you live, and on your pain relief preferences, how active you wish to be, whether you wish to use water, and whether you have a low- or high-risk pregnancy.

If your midwife or doctor does not support your choice, ask her to explain the benefits and risks to you and your baby.

At home?

Most women choose to give birth in hospital: these days it's the place to be. There is, however, evidence to suggest that if the existence of a choice was made clearer, and there was less fear of birth, more people would opt to stay at home.

If you are comfortable in your own home and you do not have a high-risk pregnancy, you may want to aim for a home birth. Women who give birth at home tend to feel more in control of their choices, less inhibited and freer to be mobile and use upright positions. Intervention is much less

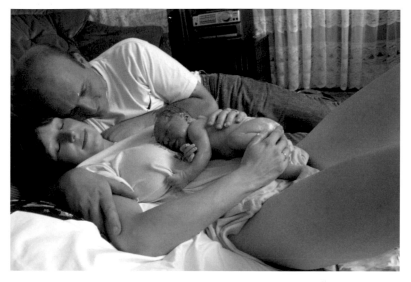

The peaceful home atmosphere is perfect for some families.

likely than in a hospital birth. This is partly because the birthing hormones flow more effectively when the environment is familiar and a woman feels relaxed and undisturbed.

Talk to your midwife about the cover for home birth that's available in your area. Your antenatal midwife may be able to come to you during labour. Having a midwife present who is like a family friend is highly rated by many couples.

Not all home births go according to plan, however, and you'll need to bear this in mind. Your midwife will monitor you and your baby, but not as closely as is possible in hospital. She is able to offer gas and air as pain relief, but not an epidural; she can perform episiotomy but not forceps or ventouse. If complications arise during or after the birth, you and your baby may need to be transferred to hospital; this happens in a minority of home births. For more information, see www.homebirth.org.uk

'It was everything that I wanted in a birth, to know that I didn't have to go anywhere. Then afterwards we just sat there and held her. We had a lovely bath together, then we snuggled into our bed, the whole family together.'
Jenny

In hospital?

All hospitals are different – they range from homely units to impersonal and unwelcoming wards. It's important to explore your own options: get a feel for the place and ask to see records of statistics including intervention, water births, use of epidural, and transfer.

On many occasions, hospital is the safest place to be – if a mother needs medical assistance, birth needs to be speeded up or a baby needs special care. There is growing evidence, however, that a high-tech medical environment and ongoing monitoring increase a mother's anxiety, raises the chance of intervention, and makes many births traumatic for mother, father and baby.

Midwifery and GP units

If you are not at high risk, you may choose a midwifery or GP unit. This may be like a home from home that you share with other women. It has similar advantages and disadvantages of a home birth and women who give birth in these 'low-risk' units celebrate a high level of satisfaction. In the unlikely event that you need further assistance and the unit is part of a larger hospital, facilities will be on hand; if the unit is an ambulance journey away from a larger hospital, this will be more disruptive.

'I couldn't have wished for a better place; the unit was fantastic, the midwives were wonderful. I enjoyed the few days after birth too, because I knew they were looking after me and they helped me learn to dress and bathe Alanah.'
Jill

Consultant-led units

If you are at high risk, or you prefer to have all facilities at hand, you will need to give birth in a consultant-led unit in a large hospital. It is not always the case, but with the option for sophisticated anaesthetics and obstetric care, disruption and intervention are more likely in this environment.

Home vs hospital: advantages and disadvantages

Home

Advantages	Disadvantages
Familiar and relaxing, freedom to move	No high-tech medical support
Continuity of care	No epidural
Higher chance of birth without intervention	Possibility of transfer to hospital in labour or after birth

Hospital

Advantages	Disadvantages
Support of medical teams in labour and after birth	You may be less free to move around; more likely to be monitored
Epidural available	More pain relief usually needed
On-site special care if you are in a teaching hospital	Higher chance of intervention
Being with other women and midwives after birth may be important for you	You may not know the midwives

'I had to go to the teaching hospital because of my blood pressure. As it was, we had no problems, and I gave birth to Gemma without any assistance. The team was fantastic, the unit was comfy. Only the food was, well, not what I would have chosen.'
Lisa

Will it go according to plan?

The majority of labours in the UK proceed without complications. There are many factors, however, that may trigger a change of plans. A complication or the need for extra caution may become apparent in pregnancy; or there may be concern during labour that necessitates a transfer. Making plans helps you to feel empowered and safe; being flexible and having a plan B will help if your expectations are not met.

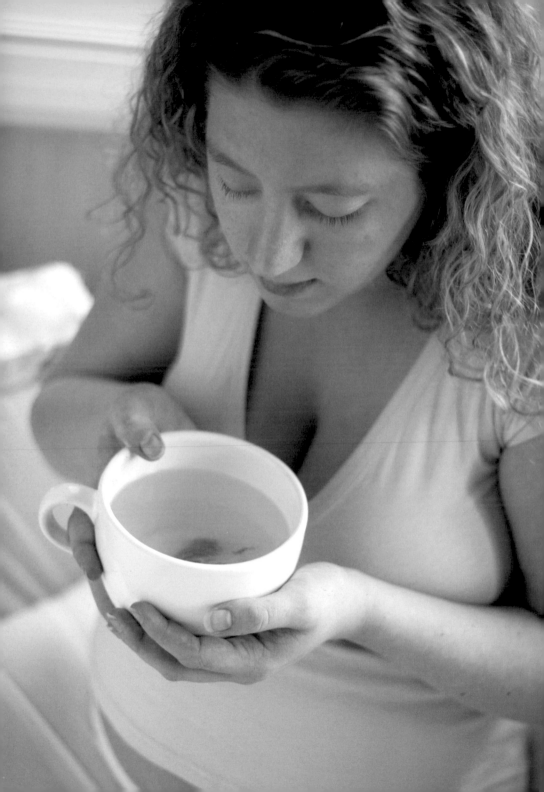

3 Week by week

There is little about being human more amazing than the miracle of growth from a single cell to a plump, crying, feeding, moving baby; or the wonder that a woman's body can nurture new life. The most intimate of relationships, wordless as it is, follows unconscious exchanges of movements, hormones and thoughts, and a pattern of physical growth that sets you and your baby up for birth. Each week takes you closer to this and your continuing union in the months beyond.

'Motherhood is the greatest gift and it deserves a happy beginning.'
Dr Gowri Motha, from *Gentle Birth Method*

Weeks 1–2

In weeks one and two there is no pregnancy but when your due date is calculated, the first week of your pregnancy will be the week of your last menstrual bleed. As your uterine lining sheds, levels of oestrogen and progesterone fall. Your brain senses this and sends out hormones from the pituitary gland that will begin a new reproductive cycle.

good to know

Your baby's genome

▶ The sperm brings 23 chromosomes, representing your partner's genetic individuality; and your egg carries its own 23 chromosomes. The combination of 46 lays down the blueprint for your baby's development.

▶ Each one of these 46 chromosomes contains around 30,000 genes.

▶ Your baby's genome is unique. It determines gender, skin colour, nose shape, and stature, as well as brain development, organ function and susceptibility to illness in later life.

▶ Increasingly precise genetic science suggests that genes also influence emotional tendencies and personality.

At the start of your reproductive cycle, follicle-stimulating hormone (FSH) stimulates a follicle on your ovary to ripen so that it can release an egg. Simultaneously, luteinizing hormone (LH) stimulates your ovaries to release more oestrogen. With balance, the follicle will ripen and release an egg at around day 14: this is ovulation. Occasionally, more than one egg is released.

The rise in oestrogen may boost your energy and sex drive. In the middle of your cycle, your body temperature rises slightly and the quality of mucus around your cervix changes: usually it forms a near-impenetrable barrier, but for three or four days it offers protection for sperm. You are ready for pregnancy.

Your egg travels into your fallopian tube. Behind it, the ruptured follicle becomes a 'corpus luteum' (yellow body). This produces progesterone to help nourish your fertilized egg for around ten weeks. The illustration on page 65 shows the egg's journey from ripening to implantation.

Your partner ejaculates as many as 300 million sperm as you make love. Only one will unite with your egg. The instant the strongest sperm reach your egg is the first decisive moment in your future baby's life. It was once thought that sperm penetrated the outer coating of the egg by releasing enzymes. Today, science suggests an egg opens its outer membrane and embraces a single sperm. Could it be that egg and sperm select each other?

Once inside, your partner's sperm sheds its tail and body and its head fuses with your egg's nucleus. The new cell that is created is called a zygote. This is the beginning of your baby.

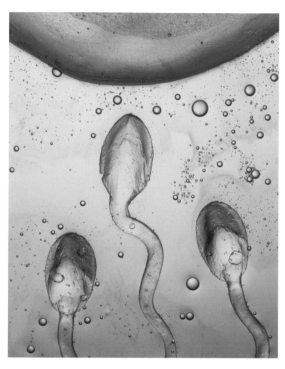

Of millions of sperm, a handful of front runners reach the egg in about 5 minutes. Behind them, back-ups are thought to deter the advances of another man's sperm.

How your baby grows

Your body adapts to provide the nutrition and protection your baby needs, and your growing baby is primed to get the very best from her womb environment. Nature works in your favour, and what you eat, how you feel, what's happening in your life also have an effect. Your baby is not fully 'programmed' like a robot ready to fulfil its purpose. Genes are exquisitely sensitive: her environment and experiences determine which genes express themselves, and when.

Weeks 3-4

The zygote that forms from sperm and egg immediately divides into two; then again – and again, and again. The resulting bundle of cells, called a 'morula' (meaning 'raspberry'), is propelled along your fallopian tube by cells in the lining, and is bathed in protective fluid.

The cells continue to divide and they group themselves around a fluid-filled centre. Roughly four days after conception, the collection of cells has grown to around 120, and has become a 'blastocyst'. It sheds its outer membrane and prepares to implant in the wall of your uterus.

Implantation, around seven days after conception, may not be smooth. Because half of the cells in the growing blastocyst come from your partner, your body recognizes them as foreign. It launches an immune attack, sending white blood cells on a mission to destroy, just as if you are harbouring a virus. Many blastocysts lose this struggle, resulting in early loss that may go unnoticed. Those that survive and implant safely on the spongy lining of the uterus are ready for the next stage: the creation of a placenta and the emergence of an embryo.

When the blastocyst makes contact with your uterus, the cells that will evolve into the placenta begin to burrow into the uterine lining to connect with your bloodstream. The other cells will develop into an embryo: at this stage they form a flat disc no bigger than a pinhead. The embryonic cells are arranged in three distinct layers:

▶ The outer layer will form your baby's neural tube, and from this her brain, spine, nervous system, skin, eyes and ears will develop.
▶ The middle layer will become her bones, muscles, heart and blood vessels.
▶ The third layer will form the other major internal organs, including her digestive system and urinary tract.
All the building blocks are in place. The cells of your uterine lining (endometrium) grow over the blastocyst to protect it.

Early signs

You may or may not have noticed a change. Often, early pregnancy symptoms seem like premenstrual feelings. You may have slightly tender breasts, urinate more frequently or be emotionally sensitive. If you have been aiming to get pregnant, the anticipation of a missed period may be enough to make you feel jittery.

Some women just 'know' they have conceived; dreams may prompt you to become suspicious. Pregnancy tests are getting more accurate and you may get a positive result now. If the test is negative, try again in a week's time: your hormone levels may not yet have altered significantly (see also overleaf).

watch out!

Spotting and implantation bleeds
Many normal pregnancies involve light bleeding or spotting in the first 12 weeks. It usually arises from blood vessels in the uterus disturbed during implantation. But as bleeding may signal a potential problem, report any blood loss to your doctor (see also page 169).

The journey of an egg, ripening, being released, meeting sperm and then, once fertilized, travelling to the safety of your uterine lining.

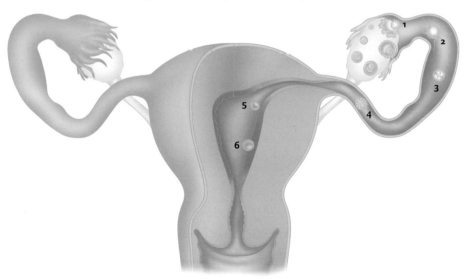

1 In your ovary, your egg ripens. It is released into your fallopian tube at ovulation (around day 14). 2 Sperm and egg meet in your fallopian tube. 3 When your egg is fertilized, a single cell develops, then divides. 4 The cells multiply to form a 'morula'. 5 Roughly four days after conception, the cluster of cells has grown to 120: a 'blastocyst'. 6 Around seven days after conception the fertilized egg implants.

Week 5

This is the time for pregnancy testing. The tests detect human chorionic gonadoptrophin (HCG), which is secreted by placental cells. You can rely on a positive result (95% accurate), but a negative result may not be correct at this early stage. Levels may not be significant until week six.

How you may feel
▶ Oestrogen begins to relax ligaments throughout your body. One of the effects may be a need to urinate more frequently, and you may feel tenderness in your breasts.
▶ Progesterone levels also rise: they support the embryo and may affect your digestive system, causing nausea and sickness, indigestion, wind or constipation. This hormone may also make you feel lethargic or tired.
▶ Both these hormones also influence your moods and can trigger vivid memories that have been hidden in your subconscious for months or even years.

Your baby
Your baby's first week as an embryo, securely protected in your uterus, is one of crucial development. The embryo is a 'C' shape. It is enclosed by two membranes and by a yolk sac, which manufactures blood cells until bone marrow forms and takes over this role. By the end of week 5, her heart has begun to form and is already beating. A tiny umbilical cord connects to the developing placenta, and minute blood vessels are in place. This is also a decisive time for brain development: neurons (brain cells) begin to double in number every 90 minutes. Specific types of cells congregate in groups to form the major brain structures. At the same time, the network of nerves in her spine and throughout her body is being established.

Week 6

The embryo inside you is taking on a 'tadpole' shape. Limb buds are forming, the brain continues its rapid development and the internal structures for the eyes, ears and nose are present.

The placental cells are multiplying, but the placenta is not yet ready to sustain your baby: the ruptured follicle on your ovary will continue to produce progesterone until the placenta matures around week 10. This progesterone release may contribute to your tiredness.

You may feel nauseous or experience 'morning sickness' which can, incidentally, occur at any time of day: this is your body's reaction to hormone changes and usually settles by weeks 10–16.

Although tiny at this stage – around 2mm (1/8in) long – your growing baby requires a great deal of nourishment. With the extra energy expenditure, you may feel hungry more often. Ideally, you need 200 extra calories a day.

Acupressure to relieve nausea

For full acupuncture treatment, visit a specialist. To help yourself, find the point 'Pericardium 6' on your wrist, two finger-widths from the meeting of your wrist and palm, in line with your middle finger. Massage the point with your thumb in an anti-clockwise direction for two minutes on each wrist, two to three times a day. Even better, get a friend or your partner to do it. Travel sickness bands, which are available from most chemists, work along this acupuncture principle.

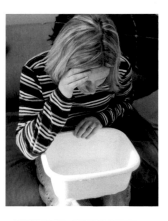

good to know

Remedies to ease nausea and sickness
▶ Of all remedies, acupuncture seems to be the most effective.
▶ Eat small quantities every two to three hours, and try chamomile and mint teas.
▶ For ginger tea, take 2–3cm (1in) fresh ginger root. Cut it into slices and simmer in 1 litre (13/4 pints) of water for 20 minutes. Strain and drink, ideally first thing in the morning. You can drink more every three to four hours. If you wish to sweeten it, add 1/2 teaspoon of honey when it has cooled a little. This drink is also wonderfully detoxifying.

Week 7

Your embryonic baby is no more than 13mm (½in) long and weighs less than 1g. Inside her body, lungs are forming, along with other organs including the liver and the beginnings of her digestive tract. The limb buds are growing and an opening that will become her mouth has appeared.

must know

Tiredness

Tiredness in the first trimester is almost universal. General fatigue may not shift until week 12–14. In the meantime:

▶ Don't worry, it's normal.

▶ Cut down on commitments where you can.

▶ Try napping during the day; resting and breathing calmly without nodding off may also be rejuvenating.

▶ Consuming coffee, sugar or other stimulants places demands on your body and in the long run will only make you more tired.

▶ An hour before bed, drink chamomile or herbal sleepy-time tea. Try to empty your bladder before falling asleep so that you won't need to get up in the night.

Your cervix is producing a thick mucus, building up a protective 'plug' that secures your uterus, keeping it separated from your vaginal canal and protected from bacteria that exist naturally in your vagina.

You may feel irritable, shocked or low, even if you are excited about pregnancy. Such feelings reflect hormonal changes and are completely normal. They are also an important aspect of your mental adjustment to pregnancy. Talking to someone you trust will help you tune into yourself, process your feelings, and move on. Telling your partner is an important part of the communication between you and will give him space to express his own feelings.

Is sex safe?

Sexual intercourse doesn't present a risk at any stage in pregnancy unless you have experienced bleeding or have a history of miscarriage: in this case, avoid intercourse for the first 14 weeks. For more on this, see pages 34-5.

Week 8

You will almost certainly notice bodily changes if you haven't already. Your uterus, softened by the action of oestrogen and progesterone and flushed with additional fluid and blood, is swelling. Your doctor will be able to feel the enlargement during an external examination. Some clothes may feel tighter.

Your uterus is now acting like a major organ. Your heart and lungs work harder than usual to deliver more blood and fluid to it and to nourish the growing placenta. The output of your heart will increase throughout pregnancy: it pumps up to 30% extra blood around your body. This is known as 'hyper-dynamic circulation'. Veins and arteries throughout your body relax to accommodate the increased flow. If you feel breathless:

▶ Make time to relax.

▶ Sit upright with a straight back – this makes space for your lungs and diaphragm.

▶ Take short moderate walks.

▶ Try yoga breathing exercises.

Meanwhile, development in the spinal cord and outer tissues allows your baby to feel touch. She is already learning about her environment.

The rapid development of nerve cells (neurones) in her brain continues. The most primitive brain regions that govern body movement and instinctive reactions are established and she has developed the 'startle reflex' (see page 83). Her nostrils appear and eyelids begin to form over her eyes (which are widely spaced). She is transforming from 'tadpole' to human shape. Your baby can be visualized with ultrasound. Vaginal scans are most accurate at this stage.

good to know

Cravings
Craving is your body telling you that it needs something. Often, cravings reflect a mineral deficiency, an unbalanced or high-sugar diet. They can also arise as a reaction to uncomfortable feelings or stress.

▶ In moderation, it's probably OK to satisfy your craving, although if you crave something that's not so good (chocolate, chips, cigarettes, whiskey or coal, for instance), it's wise not to follow your instincts.

▶ Follow the ABC (page 19) and aim for balance – in your diet, and between exercise and rest, work and play.

▶ If your cravings worry you, talk to your midwife. Advice from a nutritionist and a psychotherapist could help.

Week 9

Your baby is 10,000 times the size of the first cell formed when egg and sperm met, and 15-30mm (½-1¼in) long. Her bones are maturing and muscles are forming. She rolls and somersaults and her spine is beginning to straighten.

You may notice changes to your skin – usually it becomes plumper and softer, but it's also common to get patches of greasiness or acne. All this is due to hormonal changes. Vaginal discharge is also normal: but any bleeding needs to be investigated by your midwife (see page 169).

'My brain kept telling me I was pregnant. I thought, "Holy Shit, I can't be!". I kept ignoring it. I was nine weeks when I did a pregnancy test and found out for sure. I was gutted. I had so much planned. I'm in my 30s and Jon and I have been together for 12 years – it's like 12 years of freedom suddenly stopped. I thought – I've lost my life, I've lost me. I was grieving. When Jon came home that night he was over the moon, which made me even more gutted. We went down to the beach, I burst into tears. It was such a shock. Now I feel a lot better. I am tired but happy. I'm really excited.'
Sarah

Twins

▶ If you produce two eggs at ovulation, and each one is united with a sperm, you will have conceived non-identical twins. They have separate amniotic sacs, cords and placentas.

▶ Identical twins occur when a fertilized egg splits into two embryos. They share a placenta but dwell in separate sacs.

▶ Twins touch and explore one another via the membranes of their sacs throughout pregnancy and many enjoy continuing closeness immediately after birth.

Week 10

By the end of week ten, your baby has passed through the evolutionary phases of a fish-tadpole to mammal, and her body and brain are effectively mapped out. With this foundation in place, her body begins to take on exquisite details, like the distinction of fingers and toes and teeth buds in her gums, and her brain matures at a staggering pace.

In your baby's brain, new cells are forming at an incredible rate – at least 250,000 neurones every minute, and the rate increases each week. Neurones 'hook-up' with one another via synapses and the combination of cell division and communication gradually forms specific brain centres as well as links between them and between her brain and body. The network of synapses that takes shape through pregnancy is partly determined by her genes, and orchestrates many aspects of her development; although the precise patterns of cell groups and activity reflect her environment and what she is experiencing. Your baby's unique brain will influence her body-mind activity for the rest of her life.

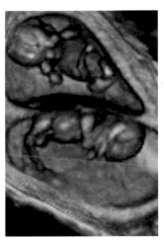

Twins at ten weeks, seen on a 3-D ultrasound scan.

'I feel pretty cool about it, I feel like a ram. It's all I can think of now. When we got the great news it was just fantastic, like yeah!'
John

Week 11

Your baby has graduated from an embryo to a foetus – derived from the Latin word meaning 'offspring'.

must know

Ulstrasound scan
The 11-week ultrasound scan is the NT or nuchal translucency scan (page 52).

The placenta is rapidly growing and by week 11 (or week 13 at the latest) replaces the corpus luteum on your ovary in progesterone production. It is your baby's companion: it breathes, excretes and digests for her, and delivers optimum nutrition, including oxygen, vitamins, essential fatty acids, glucose, minerals, antibodies and a vast range of hormones. The placenta also assists you, chiefly through its production of progesterone and oestriol hormones. Later, it plays a central role in initiating labour.

Dad
It may be difficult to engage with your baby before your partner's abdomen starts expanding; and even more so if she is tired, distracted or grumpy. Take the opportunity to learn how your baby is growing and how your partner is growing your baby. Many expectant dads find that feeling part of the process reduces the anxiety that comes with 'not knowing'.

2-D and 3-D ultrasound scans give a very different sense of a baby at 11 weeks.

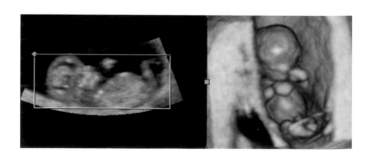

Week 12

The last week of the first trimester is often a watershed. Your uterus moves beyond your bony pelvis into your abdomen and you may feel completely different. The risk of miscarriage has now fallen significantly.

For many people, tiredness and sickness pass with as sudden a departure as their arrival weeks before. You may move into the next trimester with confidence, excitement and energy. But there are no rules, and symptoms may continue.

Inside you, your baby is twice the size she was at week nine – now plum-sized at around 60mm (2¼in) in length and weighing 13g (½oz). Her body is covered with fine downy hair and she practises breathing by taking fluid into her lungs and expelling it. She moves her limbs as she floats.

In some parts of the country, antenatal classes are heavily subscribed. Scout around and book up now, particularly if you want to attend NCT classes or specialist groups.

'When we went for the 11-week scan, I, like Jane, was very anxious. Jane had all sorts of thoughts going on in her head. I could tell just by looking at her, but when I saw the picture of this little baby, I was just blown away. It never occurred to me that as early as 12 weeks we would see a proper little baby and that the features would be clear. I looked at this baby and thought, "Oh my God, that's my child. Wow!" Then, "How am I going to support it?"'
Jason

good to know

Relief from candida
Candida is, unfortunately, more common in pregnancy. If you're affected:
▶ Relax in a warm bath infused with tea tree oil; or try calendula cream. Try homeopathy, pro-biotic (tablets or yoghurt) and echinacea.
▶ You can use over-the-counter anti-fungal cream or get it on prescription. Reserve pessaries for a moderate or severe attack.
▶ Guard against future attacks by wiping from front to back and keeping clean and dry.
▶ Keep sugar consumption to a minimum (the bacteria thrive on it).
▶ See also page 170.

Know your hormones

Hormones cause physical and emotional reactions for you and for your baby. Their levels change as part of pregnancy and in response to what's happening in your life and what you are thinking and feeling. They are vital aspects of feelings, pregnancy changes, labour and family life, for you and for your baby.

Love hormones

The 'love hormones' bring feelings of love, bliss, connection and contentment. They also reduce tension and pain: in breast milk they act more powerfully than morphine to calm a baby. Love hormones flow most strongly when you feel safe, comfortable, warm and loved, and with skin-to-skin contact.

Prolactin

This fuels your nesting instinct and urges you to focus on your baby – you may become fiercely protective. It stimulates breast milk flow and can dampen sex drive. It helps your baby feel settled and focus on you, and is important for lung development.

Oxytocin

Oxytocin rises for you and your baby through pregnancy to make you feel chilled out and loving. Oxytocin surges in the hours after birth, more so if you lie naked with your baby, and dad can boost his oxytocin buzz with skin-to-skin contact. Your baby absorbs oxytocin from your milk: love molecules on tap.

Endorphins

Otherwise known as 'feel-good hormones', these flow when you are happy, when you exercise, laugh and enjoy sexual intimacy and when you are in labour or in pain. They counteract stress and discomfort. You and your baby produce a lot during labour and dads often have endorphin rushes at birth.

Endorphin levels are boosted by a healthy immune system and rise when you're with people you love.

Oestrogen

Oestrogen rises through pregnancy to 100 times more than normal. It nourishes your uterus and relaxes your muscles, ligaments and joints; helps your vagina stay soft and moisturized; causes your breasts to swell; and increases libido. When the time is right, you, your baby and the placenta produce very high levels to stimulate contractions.

Oestrogen tends to boost wellbeing, but if it's low it can cause negative moods. The natural and dramatic fall of oestrogen after birth is one reason for 'baby blues' and postnatal depression (page 172).

good to know

Deep secrets and buried feelings
▶ Oestrogen and progesterone molecules bind themselves to areas of your brain that are important for memory, hunger, sexual desire and anger.
▶ They may awaken parts of you that have long been hidden: feelings and memories, and even recollections of your own womb life or your birth.
▶ This is often accompanied by intense emotions, especially love, awe, sadness and anger.
▶ Some women feel strongly connected to a subconscious and almost primeval maternal power.

Progesterone

Progesterone helps to soften your body and in pregnancy keeps your cervix closed. From week ten, it is produced mainly by the placenta, giving you as much as 18 times your normal levels. Before this, it comes from your ovary. Levels fall during labour, allowing your cervix to dilate. In moderate amounts, progesterone creates calm and nurturing feelings, but high levels may make you restless or anxious.

Stress hormones

Stress hormones, such as adrenaline, are a positive response to threat and are important in late labour to increase the power for birth. Your baby produces her own and picks up your stress hormones. Very high levels may make you more sensitive to pain, tense, anxious and perhaps confused. Stress hormones may run high if day-to-day life is very demanding; if your relationship(s) are tense; if you let yourself go hungry or eat lots of sugar; or if you are afraid of labour, birth or parenting. For tips on reducing stress, see page 19.

Week 13

Things begin to move on apace in the second trimester. Although every woman is different, week 13 often marks a new phase, with higher energy and optimism.

Inside your uterus, your baby may begin testing the feel of her thumb in her mouth, now that her arms are long enough. Her eyelids fuse and won't open again until the eighth month of pregnancy. On a scan, you will be able to see her features quite distinctly, although the genitals may not be discernible. She may begin to swallow the amniotic fluid, which passes through her developing kidneys and is excreted like urine.

If you haven't already visited your doctor or midwife, you need to arrange your first 'booking' visit. From now on, your midwife will want to see you every four weeks (see page 42).

Be kind to yourself
▶ Drink 2 litres (3½ pints) of room temperature water a day.
▶ Take a pregnancy multivitamin and mineral supplement, including omega fatty acids.
▶ If you're craving sweets, try fruit and nuts instead: e.g. brazil nuts, hazel nuts, pumpkin seeds. Give the change of diet a few days to take effect and then enjoy guilt-free pleasure that's really good for you and your baby.

The placenta
The placenta you and your baby share for nine months is your baby's life source, duly honoured by many midwives and mothers: you may have heard it called the baby's friend or sister. In many western hospitals, though, it is hardly mentioned.

The placenta begins to form at conception. By week 13, at the latest, it has taken over production of progesterone from your ovaries and can sustain your pregnancy. It produces hormones, growth factors and other chemicals that affect you and your baby. It is also an incredible go-between. It has tiny blood vessels, called villi, that burrowed into your uterine lining around week four. These are surrounded by cells that bathe in your blood. They absorb oxygen, protein, antibodies, haemoglobin, sugars, hormones, vitamins, minerals and fatty acids, then pass these to the placental tissue and along the umbilical cord to your baby. Waste products and hormonal messages travel the other way, from your baby to you.

The filter system is highly effective and can reject some infections and toxins; even so, most of what is in your bloodstream will be shared with your baby in pregnancy.

At week 13, the placenta is around 3cm (1¼in) in diameter. By full term, it has grown to 20cm (8in) and is around 1kg (2.2lb) in weight. It releases hormones to help trigger labour, and is born after your baby in the 'third stage' (pages 136–7). Seeing and feeling this amazing organ could be part of your birth plan. If you'd like to keep it, you could plant it under a tree. Eating it is another option and is tradition in some families. You'll find a range of recipes on the internet if you decide to serve it up. The placenta brims with goodness: some people say it boosts postnatal recovery and can reduce the chance of depression.

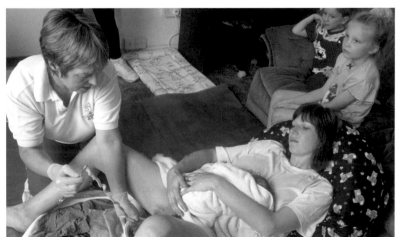

You may give birth to the placenta while you are holding your baby. Feeding your baby helps to speed up this stage of labour.

Week 14

Now that your muscles and ligaments have softened considerably, you may feel increasingly supple. Their softening is partly due to the relaxing hormone 'relaxin' and also oestrogen, and will continue through pregnancy.

You may notice your skin darkening. Usually, this happens around the nipples and areolae, and in a line from the pubis to belly button. Your face may look suntanned or develop dark patches: often most noticeable around the mouth in the 'pregnancy mask' (cloasma). These are caused by raised levels of the pigment melanin. Your skin may also take on a ruddy glow or develop small red spots as fuller blood vessels beneath the skin become visible because of extra blood and fluid in circulation. If the coloration bothers you, use natural foundation and wash your face with cool water and natural soap. In the sun, use high factor sun block (at least 50). Changes in skin tone usually pass a few months after birth.

It's OK to begin antenatal yoga and pilates, but check with your doctor and a qualified teacher that the exercises are safe for you.

As your baby's body grows, her head will begin to look more in proportion. Her facial expressions change all the time. Her fingers play with her cord and touch her body and she has room to somersault, roll

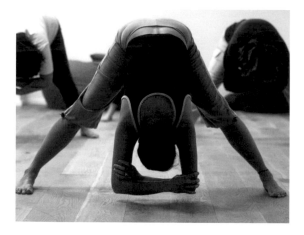

and kick. All these movements are involuntary but they are crucial for growth and, over time, contribute to your baby's awareness of her body and her watery world.

At 14 weeks, most babies are 80–110mm ($3^{1}/_{4}$–$4^{1}/_{4}$in) long from the crown of the head to the top of the legs, and around 25g (1oz) in weight.

Week 15

Your baby now hears sounds for the first time: your heartbeat and the pulsing of blood in your body; your digestion; your voice. She'll also hear some sounds in your environment, but it is the sound of you that will be most comforting when she is born.

Her skin, coated with fine downy hair (lanugo), is translucent. Her bone marrow has now matured enough to produce her blood: until now it was produced by the yolk sac. Her blood contains lymphocytes, white blood cells essential for immunity.

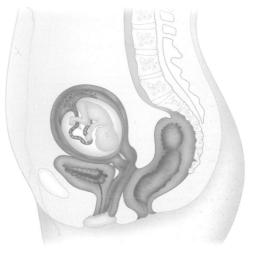

Immune cells communicate and store information so that your baby's immune system is almost like a separate brain. As nerves feed information into the bone marrow, your baby's immune system 'learns'; and it also sends information back to her brain. Her body cells and brain cells learn to recognize herself. This is the basis for growth as well as for survival. Self-knowing allows her body to respond appropriately and adapt to millions of signals every second. It will also recognize foreign matter (like bacteria or viral particles) and deal with it effectively. At this stage, your antibodies provide protection: her independent immunity develops through pregnancy and after birth.

Around the marrow, her bones are 'ossifying' or hardening. The process continues into her teenage years. She needs lots of calcium for this and will get plenty from you: your body actually absorbs more calcium than usual while you are pregnant.

Week 16

Your baby's nerves have formed enough connections for her to feel pain. She may not feel any physical discomfort in her cushioned world now, but her sensitivity means her capacity to explore explodes: and she touches the umbilical cord, feels her thumb in her mouth, fiddles with her toes and presses the walls of the amniotic sac.

Her sensitivity to taste has also increased and she can distinguish between sweet and sour: most babies prefer sweet flavours and will frown and grimace when the fluid tastes sour. If your baby is a girl, her ovaries will already contain as many as 5 million eggs – precursors of your future grandchildren.

Your baby may now weigh 80g (2¾oz) and will be up to 12cm (4¾in) from the tip of her toes to the crown of her head.

You will notice your abdomen getting gradually larger, and your breasts will also expand as they lay down fatty tissue and the milk ducts mature. You may choose to have triple tests this week (page 53).

'I woke up one morning and suddenly felt great – no more sickness, and no fatigue. Suddenly I'm buzzing around, going swimming, doing loads of walking and having sex more often, with orgasms powerful enough to move mountains. I'm enjoying my body - especially my boobs, which have blossomed from fried eggs into balloons. I can do late nights and it's quite satisfying to be the only one to wake up without a hangover. My moods are all over the place though. Jim puts up with a lot. Some nights I cry buckets for no reason I can find, others I throw "What if?" scenarios at him, moan about being fat or having greasy hair, or say that I can never be a good mum. Usually after a rant I bounce back.'
Helen

Week 17

As your baby senses more and more about herself and her environment, through sound, touch and taste, and through the chemical messages she receives from you, she forms an increasingly complex perception of life.

Within her brain, the cerebral cortex (the thinking part), which began to form in week ten, is maturing. The period between now and week 28 is really significant. By week 28, many millions of links (synapses) have been formed between neurones in the cortex to provide a basic pattern of 'wiring' that determines the way the cells interact.

This wiring will influence your baby throughout life. This early period of in-utero learning is also a time of vulnerability: external influences can be disruptive. For instance, cocaine is known to interfere with cell connections. Babies exposed to this drug in mid pregnancy are more likely to have disturbances in attention, memory, information processing and learning, as well as motor delays. Conversely, consuming essential fatty acids (see page 22) helps optimal development: EFAS are essential components of brain cells.

(see page 22)

must know

Your pelvic floor

Pregnancy is a perfect introduction to your pelvic floor, whose muscles cradle your pelvis, support your back and all the contents of your abdomen and help you to control urine flow. They soften in pregnancy (which might mean occasional and mild urinary incontinence), but getting to know them is a great way to tone them. Exercise them at least two times a day:

► Tighten your pelvic floor as if you are holding in urine. Start at the anus and gradually tighten towards your vagina.

► Tighten, count to five, consciously release, and relax. Do this five times.

► Repeat, without holding the tension.

► Choose a trigger – a soap, waiting at traffic lights, reading the paper.

► You can practice on your partner too.

► Continue daily after pregnancy: for life.

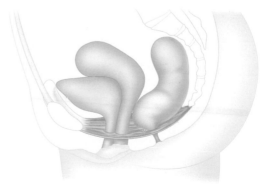

Week 18

As well as sleeping, your baby is vigorously moving and exercising. You may feel flutters: at first, the feeling may leave you wondering, but when it is repeated you'll soon be in no doubt. Don't worry if you don't feel anything – it may be week 19 or 20 before you do; and some people feel movement as early as week 15.

must know

Travelling

▶ If you're thinking of going on holiday abroad, the time between now and week 28 may be best. After this you may feel more fatigued. Most airlines don't allow women to fly beyond the 32nd week of pregnancy.

▶ Travelling in a pressurized commercial plane in pregnancy is not thought to have any detrimental effect on a baby.

▶ Make sure you drink plenty of water to avoid dehydration.

▶ To guard against swelling and deep vein thrombosis (DVT), wear support tights throughout the flight, and walk around every one or two hours to keep your circulation going.

▶ To reduce blood clotting, especially if you have varicose veins (page 186), you can safely take a 75mg, low-dose aspirin before you set off; you could use homeopathic Arnica (30c or 200c) if you prefer.

Posture

Your posture will change naturally as your abdomen grows and your spine softens and curves. How you stand and sit will also affect your energy, the sensations of digestion and sensitivity to pain, and good posture can help to tone your muscles. These tips could help your pregnancy run more smoothly:

▶ Use chairs that support your back and place your feet flat on the floor or a low foot rest. Try to avoid crossing your legs.

▶ Sit on the floor with your back supported and a cushion under your bottom in preference to slouching on a sofa.

▶ When you stand, let your feet take your weight equally and try not to let your pelvis fall forward. Keep your chin down to reduce strain in your neck and spine.

▶ Invest in a supportive mattress. Using pillows between your thighs, under your hips or under your knees helps to reduce pelvic and back pain.

▶ Regular yoga (see page 30) or pilates will help tone your muscles and improve posture.

Week 19

You'll be able to notice your baby's incredible growth by the increasing size of your abdomen. By this week nervous connections have formed between your baby's muscles and her brain and some scientists believe that this allows conscious direction of movements.

Your baby will have grown to between 12 and 14cm (4³/₄ and 5¹/₂in), from her bottom to the top of her head, and will weigh around 150g (just over 5oz). If you have a scan this week, you can get accurate measurements.

'Sex is still good if slightly less animated and frequent. I'm not too bothered about hearing about other people's experiences and try to avoid practical parenting conversations – plenty of time for that later, as it is a bit dull. I was worrying about the future and I have been searching for a plan, preparing for some self-sacrifice if need be. Fortunately, fate smiled on us and I don't have to worry too much.'
Mark

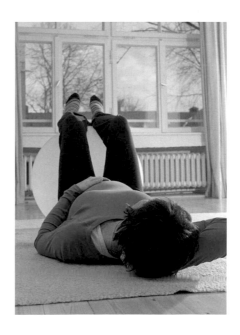

A perfect pose for relieving tension or back pain 15 minutes in this position with your head on a pillow is relaxing and refreshing, and relieves back ache. Don't do it in late pregnancy if it's uncomfortable. After birth, you can lie your baby on your chest or stomach.

Week 20

Your partner and any other curious people may now be able to feel kicks by laying their hands on your abdomen. Your baby may be most active when you relax, perhaps as you lie in the bath or when you are in bed.

must know

What sex is your baby – to know or not to know?
If you have your heart set on one sex, the 20-week scan can reveal it. If your hopes are dashed, you will have time to get used to the idea. Disappointment about gender can contribute to postnatal blues and affect bonding: recognizing your feelings and talking about them now could be positive for all of you.

Inside your abdomen, even though her eyelids are still fused, your baby can sense changes in light: if you flash a light on your abdomen, she will notice. You might feel a movement in response.

'I am being as supportive as I thought I could be but it's a bit of a tightrope sometimes. As most men will agree, women can be prone to bouts of emotional turbulence, to say the least. H is growing more lovely the more she grows our baby. She isn't so tired and has stopped being sick, she looks pregnant and happy. Going for scans is a nice experience and it has brought us closer together – visual proof of impending parenthood. It moved, it moved, and then I try and feel, but miss it.'
David

Music
Any sounds your baby hears during pregnancy add to her memory. The most significant thing is how much you enjoy music (if you love it, your baby will share your 'feel good' endorphin hormones), and if you dance, even better for both of you. There may be some truth in the rumour that classical music is good for babies. Music with a rhythm of 55–70 beats per minute, for instance, stimulates relaxed 'alpha' brain waves and reduces stress. Mozart is a popular choice.

Week 21

Your baby is laying down insulating fat and a special fatty substance (myelin) to coat the nerves running through her brain and body. She is also producing a white, waxy substance from the sebaceous glands in her skin. This is vernix caseosa, which protects her skin. You will notice it on her body at birth.

You may already be making preparations – planning the nursery, considering pushchairs, cots, sleeping bags and so on. This is often where expectant dads feel involved: buying a car seat that fits well, choosing monitors and other electrical gadgets, and doing DIY tasks that mums need to avoid (like paint stripping). Other ways for your partner to be part of the action include massaging you. Try tangerine oil, which is a good all-rounder to reduce aches and pains, improve sleep, calm leg cramps and lift your mood. Return the favour for him

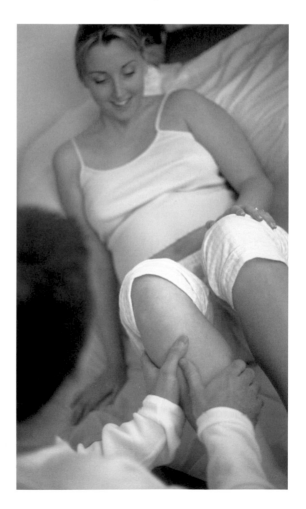

Massage is pleasurable for giver and receiver alike, and can deepen intimacy. Be sure never to massage directly over any varicose veins.

Week 22

Week 22 is something of a milestone for your baby. By this stage, most of the cell growth in her brain is complete. Billions of neurones are in place – many more than she will ever use. From now on brain development centres on the forging of links between cells. Most of these links form because of experience.

The brain is not a system of wires like a computer, even though the term 'wiring' is used to describe the connections between cells. Nevertheless, cells that work together repeatedly are more likely to fire together in the future. In this way, patterns of brain activity form. Your baby learns through touch, noises, smell and taste, from her movements and body sensations, and from the way you move, speak and feel emotionally. As her experiences are repeated, she learns to recognize and to predict. She develops skills, such as sucking, and comes to expect things. For instance, she learns to recognize the lilting tone of her 'mother tongue' and after birth she will tune into your voice most keenly.

Welcoming the spirit
Baby's spirit or soul – has it arrived? Some people believe it settles in around this week. Some energy therapists claim to be able to feel the shift and the influence of a baby's soul energy on a mother: some mothers feel it too. Is it significant that an ancient view on the emergence of individuality and a modern neuro-scientific view of brain development and learning ability both pinpoint week 22 as a crucial time?

'My partner has been doing loads of reading, he wants a home birth. We hope to have the birth in Dominica in the house where I grew up. As long as I let my obstetrician know I feel empowered, there shouldn't be a problem. I want to do it just with my partner – I think it will be a mind-blowing experience. I don't think birth should be associated with sickness, that's something that's got to change.'
Emma

Week 23

Your baby may now weigh almost 500g (around 1lb) and may be 20cm (8in) in length from crown to rump. You'll feel movements more strongly and sometimes you may notice small, rhythmic jumps as she hiccups.

By now your baby is adept at swallowing and uses the salt and sugar content of the amniotic fluid to supplement the nutrition she gets from you, via the placenta. Her sucking reflex is strong, and she may suck for long periods on her thumb. As her nerve and skin sensitivity increase, she'll spend more time stroking her umbilical cord, brushing against the amniotic sac, and exploring her body with her hands. She can also be soothed by the sensations she gets when you stroke and rub your uterus.

Throughout pregnancy, the muscles of your uterus have been contracting. The alternating tightening and relaxing is getting stronger now and you may experience your first Braxton-Hicks contractions. They are also called 'practice' contractions. These are seldom painful and usually come in short runs, intermittently. Some days you may not notice them. They are probably soothing for your baby, like a massage, and build up your muscle strength in preparation for labour.

Use only natural oils on your skin: it's so absorbent that if you rub garlic on your foot, it will be on your breath in less than an hour.

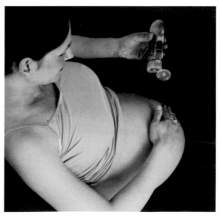

Week 24

An ultrasound at this stage, particularly 3-D ultrasound, will reveal your baby's face almost exactly as it will look at birth. All of her features are fully formed and in proportion and she will have hair on her scalp, eyebrows and eyelashes.

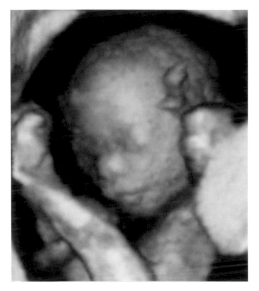

A baby seen at 24 weeks on a 3-D ultrasound scan, lying 'feet up', with eyelids still fused.

Your baby's size now limits movement inside your uterus, so although she will still kick, wriggle and reach out her hands, and can slowly turn, she can no longer somersault.

As your uterus enlarges, you may feel a little uncomfortable, particularly at night. Use extra pillows to support your bump, and a pillow between your legs if you have pelvic discomfort.

From week 24, gestational diabetes, a form of diabetes specific to pregnancy, sometimes becomes apparent. It may give symptoms such as dizziness and comes on because the action of insulin is affected by pregnancy-related hormones. If you are affected, find out more on page 173.

'My greatest support is my husband. I probably don't give him enough recognition and friendship, in fact almost definitely! He has been really excited, and more and more so. Now he's beside himself waiting to meet the baby – he wants to catch the baby!'
Isobel

Week 25

Now that your uterus is taking up more of your abdomen, you may need to reduce meal sizes. Many women get acid reflux. It will be exacerbated if you eat too much and it might help to eat small amounts slightly more frequently and avoid acidic foods like oranges. (For more, see Indigestion, page 176.)

If you are working, make sure you have made clear arrangements for maternity leave. To qualify for your entitlements, you are legally obliged to have informed your employer by this stage (see page 32).

You will have been aware of your baby's movements for a number of weeks. Around week 25 you may begin to notice patterns as your baby settles into her own rhythm, moving from waking to deep sleep, light, restless sleep, and dream sleep. Sleep is just as important for her as it is for you: it is a time for rest and involves brain wave patterns that help her consolidate all she is learning and continue to develop optimally.

Your baby has by now mastered the 'righting reflex' – a response to gravity and to your movements that might contribute to her movement into a head-down position later in pregnancy.

Feeling blue

It may not often be talked about, but feeling blue in pregnancy is common. Hormonal changes affect your moods, your partnership is adapting and there are many things to consider in the run up to birth. Feeling low, afraid or confused is normal and you are not doing anything 'wrong' if you don't feel blooming and excited. Confide in people you love and trust. Looking at your feelings is an important part of the journey of parenthood. Take time to do things that make you feel good and follow the ABC (page 19).

good to know

Lavender oil
From now on, it's safe for you to use lavender oil in the bath or mixed with a carrier oil for massage.

Week 26

This is the last week of the second trimester. Your baby will have grown to around 23cm (9¾in) and may now weigh 900g (2lb). Her wrinkly skin is beginning to appear smoother as more fat is laid down, and the lanugo hair over her body may become thinner.

Her eyelids unfuse, now that her retinas are fully formed. She will open her eyes to look out into the darkness around her. If light is shining on your abdomen, her world will appear red and watery.

In the womb your baby won't get any practice looking on distant objects, but she is able to focus. The ideal focal length for her eyes is the distance between your breast and your face: when you hold her to your chest in the moments after birth she will be able to see your features very clearly. This is wonderful genetic programming: your baby will be adept at catching your eye and learning to recognize you. As you make eye contact, the bond between you grows. There are some scientific facts accounting for this magic: eye contact activates genes in baby and adult, which trigger the release of hormones that boost feelings of love, happiness and connection.

If your partner gets close in pregnancy, your baby senses him. At birth, she will recognize his energy and his touch, and the tone and melody of his speech.

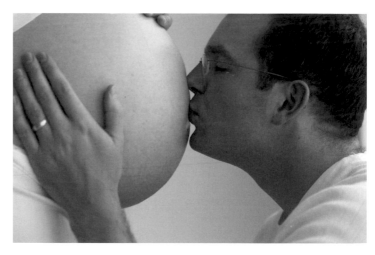

Visualization

You visualize all the time: what may happen tomorrow, what others may be doing, or what's happened in the past. With each imagining, thoughts and feelings stimulate your nervous and hormonal systems, your cells and even your genes.

Athletes often use visualization to prepare. It does more than boost confidence: visualization puts body and mind through a 'dress rehearsal'. Even though your body isn't moving, beneath your skin, nerves fire and genes respond to your thoughts. The more you rehearse, the more effortlessly you will perform when the time comes. You can use visualization to relax and/or to prepare for birth. It could also be useful for your birth partner in labour. Take your time. Turn off the phones, get comfortable and warm, sit or lie down, relax and calm your breathing.

Relaxing
Imagine yourself in a restful, warm place: tension falls away. Imagine you can see blood, oxygen, fluid and feel-good hormones flowing as your muscles soften and relax. Take your attention into your pelvis. Visualize your muscles and ligaments softening as your pelvis opens, ready for birth. Your baby floats peacefully, is gently massaged and hears the sounds of your body. Towards the end of pregnancy, invite your baby to prepare herself for birth.

Birth preparation
Visualize your cervix gradually ripening, becoming softer and stretchier in the last few weeks. Take yourself, stage by stage, through a gentle birth, with your womb tightening and relaxing, your vagina and pelvis opening and your baby pushing on your cervix and then travelling downwards. Picture yourself riding through pain, see yourself as a powerful woman working in unison with your baby towards birth. For more information, see Dr Gowri Motha's *Gentle Birth Method* and www.jeyarani.com for audio tapes and tips.

Lessons in life

Your womb is your baby's classroom. Each cell is a tiny sensory organ that picks up information, internalizes it, and responds. She experiences, explores and learns.

By now, your baby is adept at swallowing and she practises 'breathing' by drawing fluid into her lungs and passing it out. Because she sucks she's ready to suck at your breast; she also recognizes your voice. She 'rehearses' facial expressions that will engage your attention and show her feelings.

She also picks up your emotions, which are reflected in every event in your body, including your hormones, voice, heartbeat and the neurotransmitters that flow with your thoughts. She learns to associate feelings, sensations and movements. By the time she is born, what she has learnt will help her to thrive and will affect the way she behaves after birth.

Developing: on cue and in situ

Every human being is genetically programmed to develop in certain ways but it's not all pre-set: our genes actually re-programme themselves to adapt to the environment. In the uterus, development reflects how we experience life in the womb and our parents' lives beyond the womb.

Your baby, like every human, establishes patterns of gene and cell behaviour and brain activity that, like a recording, play on and on or are repeated when a familiar situation arises. This is essential – without patterning she could not breathe, co-ordinate her limbs, eat, speak or learn. It's also key to her personality. What happens in pregnancy, birth, and in the precious period that follows, lays foundations that influence your baby's entire life. There is no right or wrong: forming patterns is the way that humans adapt, learn and survive.

Emotional intelligence

For your baby, life is measured in emotional and physical sensations. In the womb, she can feel comfortable, loved, stressed or angry. Outside your womb, she will continue to have a rich emotional life, and may show responses she developed in pregnancy such as curling into a ball or kicking out if she senses danger, or sucking her hand when she's relaxed.

You cannot control your baby's emotions but even in pregnancy you have some influence in her emotional experience and what she learns about feelings. If you're stressed, for instance, relax and tell her what you're feeling, let her know that these are not her feelings, that it is not her fault: you alter the chemical messages that travel to her and you are building a foundation for acceptance and honesty. As you let her know you accept her, you are meeting one of her most basic emotional needs and will foster her sense of security and self-esteem. This may be unconscious, but nervous links within and beyond the brain are all significant in the flowering of her emotional intelligence.

After birth, your baby's experiences build on what she has reaped in pregnancy and she continues to develop emotionally as well as physically in response to her environment and her family. The sensitivity of the first year is thought to be a hugely significant foundation for 'emotional intelligence' through life – self-esteem, how it feels to be loved, to be angry or sad, and personal body image.

'The ideal environment for any baby is a loving, safe, welcoming, accepting and respectful womb. You can begin to create this by taking time for yourself, noticing how you are feeling, communicating your feelings consciously with your baby, and most importantly taking responsibility for any stress or negative feelings and getting support with them. Acknowledge his or her existence with joy, trying not to place conditions on him or her, for all babies are individuals in their own right: the more you delight in your baby, the more she will delight in herself.'
Kitty Hagenbach, mother and psychotherapist

Week 27

This week marks the beginning of the third trimester of your pregnancy. There is often a growing sense of expectation. You may now begin counting down to the birth, rather than counting up from conception.

With each week your abdomen will enlarge. Your breasts are also growing as the milk ducts mature, and they may feel tender. Your baby's rapid brain development continues, partly following her genetic tendency, and partly responding to her environment. She is constantly exposed to your emotional, physical and mental state as your hormones, neurotransmitters and other chemicals travel to her. She experiences the sound of your voice and others voices in this wider context, and begins to associate tone and volume with emotions.

If you are avoiding finding out about labour, try not to put it off. It may be daunting, but being informed can help to reduce anxiety, boost your sense of control and confidence, and could improve progress on the day. You can read, watch videos, listen to tapes and talk to other parents. It's just as important for your birth partner to get informed: this could boost his confidence and help him to feel useful during labour and a part of the process. An important aspect of his role may be as a go-between for you and the midwives and doctors.

You may attend your first antenatal class around this week. It is rare for babies to be born at week 27 (13 weeks premature), but it can happen. Fortunately, modern medical advances mean that many babies born at this age survive and thrive (see Premature labour and birth, page 181).

Week 28

Now around 25cm (10in) from crown to rump and over 1kg (2.2lb) in weight, your baby is really beginning to fathom out her world. In her brain, the cortex – the centre for thought and reasoning – is incredibly active. It is organizing all the information coming from her developing organs and senses.

Every single experience is registered within the neuro-filing cabinet that consists of around 200 billion cells, each of which may connect with hundreds or thousands of others. By week 28, your baby is already able to recognize your voice and to anticipate the melody of your speech, and she will also settle or become active to familiar music. For you, antenatal care starts to increase. You may begin to see your midwife and/or obstetrician every two weeks. If you have started antenatal classes, you'll be meeting other expectant mums and dads: some may become your friends over the next few months.

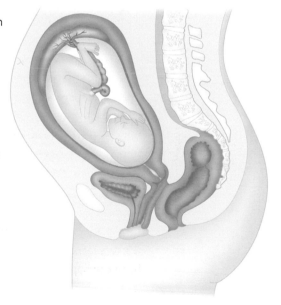

'It's amazing how much nature's there already with the baby – so much character there. It's inside me now, all forming. I love my bump. It's not a spiritual thing. It is a connection of energy. I give my baby energy and my baby gives me energy.'
Jenny

Week 29

Around week 29 you may begin to feel the urge to tidy and get things ready. If you are at work, you may be feeling less interested in your job. Quite rightly, you are focusing more on your baby and the birth you both await. Doing anything else may be frustrating and draining.

Your state of mind is partly fuelled by the hormone prolactin, which you produce increasingly from now on. Your baby helps your body produce this hormone by sending her own chemical into your system, via the placenta. Prolactin also helps your breasts to produce milk and you may notice a watery fluid leaking from your breasts. This is colostrum, which is packed with goodness and will flow for two to three days after birth until your milk comes in. Not all women experience colostrum leakage.

If you are carrying twins, they may be born early. While the average birth date for twins is week 37, they may arrive from week 28 onwards. A baby's lungs are not fully matured at this stage of pregnancy so if birth is premature, steroid hormones are used to speed up lung development and artificial ventilation may be needed for some time. Premature birth is a shock for mother, father and baby. It takes time to get used to the environment of a special care baby unit (SCBU) and parents are naturally concerned about their babies. For more, turn to page 182.

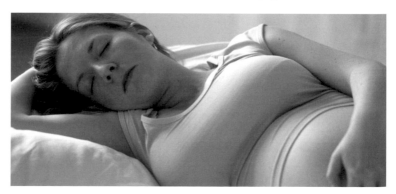

Week 30

You may be feeling slower now and, at times, clumsy or absent-minded. So don't forget to put your feet up – literally. This will help prevent fluid pooling in your ankles, which can cause swelling and faintness.

You can use week 30 as a turning point. With just ten weeks to go, labour may feel close but you have time to prepare and to enjoy the remainder of your pregnancy. Your partner may feel more engaged now you are larger, and with birth getting closer he may be more interested in how he can be involved. Finding out the facts – and the fictions – together could be fun and useful. You'll discover you both have anxieties and expectations. With these out in the open, making plans will be more enjoyable.

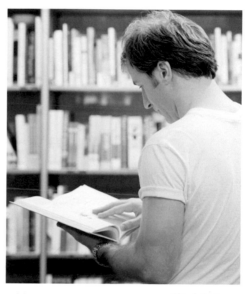

Slowly but surely, information aimed at expectant fathers is growing.

'It's quite hard sometimes, standing on the side lines. I bit the bullet and said I'd go to antenatal classes. Fortunately, there were other men there. At first we stuck to our partners' sides, but there's a couple of guys I talk to at the end of the classes now. It's reassuring to be with other men who've never been through this before. It's a relief, too, to talk about things that have nothing to do with babies. In the classes I've found out quite a bit about what tends to happen and some of the positions Fiona might want to take. I like the breathing exercises. I can't say I'm any less nervous, though. I am pretty squeamish.'
Robin

Week 31

From week 31 the sacs in your baby's lungs begin producing a substance that is called surfactant, which will help her breathe in air. Her lungs will continue to mature over the coming weeks ready for birth.

Physically, she needs to lay down more insulating body fat, but apart from this the most intense development involves her nerves, which are firing rapidly throughout her brain and body. In her brain, the learning is most intense. Even in her sleep millions of neurones fire at an incredible rate.

Inverted or flat nipples

If your nipples are flat against your areolae or go in, rather than out, don't panic. This does not usually interfere with feeding. If they have not protruded by week 35, you can begin to coax them outwards. Try gentle pressure, with your fingers underneath each areola and your thumb on top and gently press and push back towards your chest. Start delicately to allow your nipple skin to soften. You can also use a thimble-like device made by breast pump manufacturers to help your nipple protrude before a feed. Or you can try a breast shell with a hole for the nipple that gives gentle suction. Anything you use after birth must be sterilized.

Stem cells

Stem cells are found in embryos and in the blood of the umbilical cord and can, in theory, develop into any bodily tissue. The science behind the use of stem cells to replace or repair damaged body tissues months or years after birth, or in a close family relative, is still in its infancy. There is no way to say for certain whether the anticipated benefits – such as using stem cells to treat Parkinson's disease – will become a reality. If you want to store cells from the cord after birth, you'll need to plan this in advance. Find out more at www.midwivesonline.com/cells4life2.htm and www.stemcellforum.org.

Week 32

You've lost your keys again, or found them in the fridge, missed that dental appointment and forgotten your mum's birthday? Don't worry – confusion and forgetfulness are extremely common at this stage of a pregnancy.

There are many explanations, varying from the hormone oxytocin reducing electrical activity in some brain regions, to different sleep patterns. 'Cheese brain' is normal and can strike at any time. It may, however, be exacerbated if you're doing too much. You may need to reduce the amount you commit to. If circumstances make this hard, do ask for and accept help to reduce your load.

It may help to write lists, but be sure to keep them somewhere you can see them (not under a pile of magazines). Try the three-column approach – urgent, important and preferable – and tick things off as you go: it's a good feeling. You can do it with your partner or at least stick it up where he can see it. He may help you organize tasks more effectively, and remind you what you are committed to. Remember to include on your list 'time for me', 'rest' and 'time for us'.

Your baby is probably oblivious to your own mental fuzziness. Around week 32 she will have grown to roughly 29cm (11½in) from the top of her head to her bottom, and will weigh around 1.8kg (4lb).

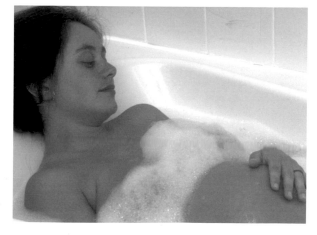

Your baby may move vigorously as you relax in the bath.

Week 33

Your baby is more cramped now, but still has room to move. Here are a few tips on helping her take a good position for birth and reducing your own discomfort.

Do

▶ Sit upright with your back supported, allowing your baby space to move.

▶ Spend time each day on all fours or kneeling and leaning forward to encourage your baby to lie towards your abdomen instead of your spine.

▶ Do yoga (see page 30) and recommended antenatal exercises.

▶ Go for walks and/or swim.

▶ Try a pregnancy rocker chair or upright kneeler, which supports your spine and allows you to rest with your knees forward.

▶ Sleep on your side with your top knee resting forwards, or on a pillow – this creates a hammock for your baby.

Don't

▶ Slouch on a soft chair or sofa. In this position, your baby may find it most comfortable to lie with her back towards your spine in occipito posterior position (page 107).

▶ Take long car journeys if the seat doesn't support upright sitting.

▶ Sit cross-legged for long periods, which reduces space – open your legs wide instead.

▶ Squat until week 38 or 39. If you squat a lot before this time and your baby is already lying awkwardly, she may be encouraged to drop down into your pelvis and then it will be more difficult for her to change position.

Remember: you can only influence your baby's position, you cannot control it – your body, her body and the position of the placenta all play a role. Sometimes a position that seems awkward for birth is actually best for a baby. For more information, see *Optimal Foetal Positioning* by Jean Sutton and Pauline Scott.

Week 34

Your baby is almost 2.25kg (5lb) and as long as 32cm (over 12in). She has shed most of the downy hair that covered her body but is still covered in creamy vernix.

Her sense of taste is at its height – more active now than at any other time of her life. She knows the taste of you. The areolae around your nipples secrete a substance that scientists believe tastes and smells almost exactly like amniotic fluid. She will be powerfully drawn towards your breasts after birth for emotional comfort and for nutrition.

good to know

Lung maturity
If your baby is born now her lungs may be mature enough to allow her to breathe without extra assistance.

IQ and EQ

Believe it or not, a prenatal university was set up in California by obstetrician Rene Van de Carr. Lessons start around week 20. Parents push on the abdomen when they feel their baby move, and babies often respond with accuracy: one kick for one push, two for two pushes, and so on. Lessons also involve repeating words like 'pat' and 'rub' while performing the action on the abdomen. Findings suggest that after birth responsive babies are more attentive and even perform better in schools.

Whether IQ can be built in the womb is not certain: but a baby who is involved in communication before birth may well be more attentive afterwards. As long as you aren't driven by expectations of high achievement, the nurturing effect of talking and listening could be profound. It certainly supports family bonding and emotional intelligence (EQ).

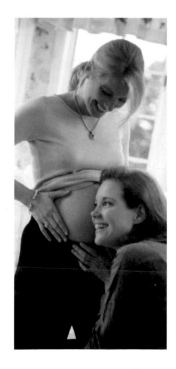

Week 35

Your baby is alert, responsive and active, even though she has less free space. Her rooting reflex – important for locating your nipple after birth – has developed. You and she are in constant communication via chemical molecules, through movement, through intuitive senses and in dreams.

good to know

Raspberry ripeness
Raspberry leaf tea is a tonic for your uterus. You'll find this in a health food shop and from various internet stockists. Don't drink it before week 36; but from week 36 you can drink it twice a day.

Try to fit regular antenatal exercises into each day if you haven't already (see pages 28–31). Focus on exercises that allow you to deepen your breathing and open your pelvis.

Premature rupture of the membranes (PROM)
If your waters break before Week 37, this is known as PROM. Around 3–5% women experience this. If it happens, you may experience a gush of clear fluid, perhaps with a little blood mixed in it; sometimes the leak is barely noticeable and may be mistaken for heavy discharge or urine leaking. Amniotic fluid is clear, watery and sweet smelling.

Once the waters have broken, labour usually begins spontaneously within 24 hours. If PROM occurs before week 35, the risks associated with prematurity are greater and you may be kept in hospital and given medication to delay labour. If leakage is minimal, you may be able to return home to rest and because your baby constantly makes amniotic fluid, her environment may not be compromised.

You must tell your doctor/midwife and go to hospital, where the loss will be assessed and a swab taken to check for vaginal infection, and your baby will be assessed using ultrasound. If an infection is detected, antiobiotics are usually given and early birth may be advised. After birth, some doctors recommend antibiotics without a blood test, but you do have the right to request a test if you wish to avoid giving your baby unnecessary antibiotics.

Week 36

You have entered the last month and you may feel very large and heavy. Take it easy and eat small meals at close intervals to keep your energy up without overloading your stomach.

From week 36 it is safe to begin massaging your vagina. This has been practised for centuries in India and Africa, and gradually increases the ease with which your muscles will stretch. If your vagina stretches well, there is less risk of tearing and of bruising. It's also good to know that you have prepared your vagina: a psychological prop that may reduce anxiety.

The best position is to prop one foot up on a chair or the bath, and reach into your vagina from behind. Alternatively, your partner could do it while you sit with your back at an angle of around 45 degrees.

▶ Wash your hands.

▶ Take a minute to calm your breathing.

▶ Insert one finger, up to the first knuckle, into your vagina.

▶ Breathe in deeply and, as you exhale, gently press your finger back towards your coccyx (your 'tail bone' at the very base of your spine). Repeat rhythmically, releasing pressure as you breathe in and pressing down gently as you breathe out. (You are training your tissues to give as you exhale in labour.)

▶ After six exhalations, change the direction of pressure to the left. After another six, change to the right. Focus only on these three areas: it is as if the back of your vagina is 12 o'clock, the right is 2 o'clock and the left 10 o'clock.

▶ Do this once a day. By the end of the first week you may feel more give in your vagina. When you are ready, insert two fingers, just up to the first knuckle. After another week, you can try to insert two fingers up to the second knuckle.

'Ask someone to paint your toe nails for you.'
Suzie

Week 37

Congratulations! At week 37 your pregnancy is considered to be full term. Your baby could be born any day. If you haven't prepared what you need for the birth, now's the time to do it. Think about what you would like to have with you for comfort in labour and revise, or create, your birth plan (pages 114–15).

Occipito anterior. **The most efficient position – it's easiest for your baby to descend. Her back may be to the left or right.**

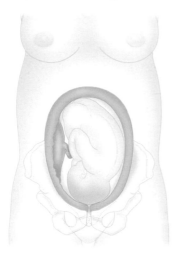

You and your baby are getting ready for labour and you might notice some of the changes to your body and your state of mind. Braxton-Hicks contractions may become stronger and more regular. Your cervix gradually softens so that is ripe enough to open when true contractions begin. At the same time, the milk ducts in your breasts are reaching maturity. Your nipples and areolae may have enlarged considerably.

Most babies take their final position for birth by week 37, although some do move in the last couple of weeks. Your baby's position depends on her size and shape and the size and shape of your pelvis. There are, broadly speaking, four main positions, illustrated here and on pages 105, 106 and 107.

If your baby is head down (and most are), you'll feel strong kicks in your rib cage. You may also feel a 'lightening' if your baby's head engages in your pelvis. Your midwife can measure the extent of engagement by feeling your uterus.

Many couples feel more intimate in the last month. There may also be anxiety: all your feelings – joy, hope, fear and sadness – are integral to your transition as parents.

Week 38

You may notice that your weight has stopped rising. This can happen even though your baby is continuing to lay down fat beneath her skin. Some women actually lose a few pounds in the last month.

If you are becoming tired, it is important to rest as much as you need to in order to enjoy each day. Remember, this includes rest without sleep – enjoying a book, some films or music, or doing some visualizations (page 91) or resting with your partner. Exercise will improve the quality of your rest: maybe a walk each day and some antenatal exercises or yoga.

If your baby's head has moved into your pelvis by now, you may need to urinate more frequently and have small leaks of urine (for more information, see page 176).

If your baby is in breech position

Your baby has probably chosen the best position but if you want to try to turn her to ease labour, the most effective way is to have a series of acupuncture treatments with moxa herbs. This must, however, be done precisely by a practitioner who has a proven track record: some have success rates of 70%. The medical technique known as ECV (external cephalic version) is less effective but can work. It must be done by a consultant obstetrician with ultrasound guidance.

must know

Caesarean section
If you have elected to have a caesarean, you may be booked to have it this week (see page 142).

Breech. **With her head up and her bottom down, your baby is in the most tricky position for vaginal birth. Most hospitals recommend caesarean delivery.**

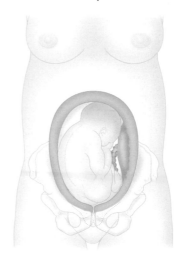

Week 39

Your baby is fully mature and busy growing and laying down fat.
She is aware of all the sounds around her and may relax to your
voice or if you play familiar music.

Squatting

This is a great form of exercise for
this week as well as taking a walk
each day. You can use a birth ball
or a low stool, or hold onto your
partner's hands or the back of a
chair (page 119). It is good
practice for labour and
strengthens your calves and
thighs. It also opens your pelvis
and encourages your baby's head
to press on your cervix,
persuading it to ripen. If your
midwife tells you your baby is in a
posterior position (page 107) but
not yet engaged, don't squat.

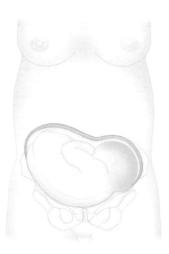

You may notice patterns to her activity, with most
movement when you rest. The rocking motion of
your body as you walk will probably soothe her, and
she will also be feeling gently massaged by Braxton-
Hicks contractions. To some extent, your baby's
patterns reflect your activity but they are also part of
her uniqueness. She moves from wakefulness to
sleep in a pattern regulated by her own 'clock genes',
and this will continue after birth. Other clock genes
affect nervous activity and ensure restful periods
where her body absorbs information and learns.
Dreaming is an important part of this.

Check the movements

Mothers often feel fewer kicks in the last week or
two of pregnancy. This is normal but because foetal
movement is a good sign, remain aware. When you
have counted ten, you can stop counting. If you
notice fewer than ten in a 24-hour period, move
around a little, eat something and be observant for
another hour. If you still feel few movements, call
your doctor. Absence of movement may mean your
baby is sleeping, but could be a sign of foetal
distress: if there is foetal distress it may be safest for
your baby to be born.

Transverse lie. **Your baby is lying across your abdomen.
Caesarean section delivery is essential.**

Week 40

Week 40 is the magic week, the week your baby is officially 'due'. Yet the due date is always a guestimate. Only four in every 100 babies arrive on the day they are expected. Labour will start when both you and your baby are ready. Your baby plays a hugely important role and at every stage you are both equally involved.

You are probably hyper-alert to unusual signs now. You may feel excited or nervous, or both! It's very common now (and earlier) to feel fed up with being pregnant. Waiting may dominate every moment and make you absent-minded. Spend some time each day sitting with your hands on your abdomen and focusing on your baby: ask her if she is ready. You might want to talk to her about the imminent birth.

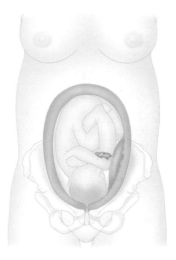

'I began to think a lot about who this baby would be, and how it might change our lives. I became quite internal and would spend hours just sitting looking at the garden or the clouds passing overhead. My brain wasn't actually much good for anything else. I had a passion for making puddings but most were disastrous and one took me three days (also disastrous). Thought I would certainly be early, 'cos I was so huge, but the due date passed. Tried sex (funny when you're like a hippo mounting a mule), Chinese food (more indigestion) and squatting. No signs – this baby didn't want to leave!'
Jeannie

***Occipito posterior*. With her back towards your spine, it might be more difficult for your baby to flex her head as she descends. Your contractions may give mostly back pain. Spend time on your hands and knees, weeding, cleaning or in yoga postures, in the last few weeks – this may encourage her to turn.**

Week 41 plus

So, your due date came and went, and you're still waiting. Don't worry, this often happens and is very common in first pregnancies. Your midwife will ask you to see you at week 41. She may invite you back for another visit at week 42; or you may want to consider induction before this.

Why induce?

Beyond week 41 your placenta may begin to function less efficiently. Placental function and your baby can be checked with ultrasound. If placental function appears to be compromised, unless you require a caesarean, induction will be recommended. Medical induction may not be recommended if your baby is in an awkward position or if you have had previous abdominal surgery. If your placenta is functioning well and your baby is thriving, you may still consider induction if:

▶ You are really fed up with being pregnant.

▶ There are physical considerations, such as high blood pressure or pronounced discomfort.

▶ Your baby is large, particularly if you have had a large baby in the past or if you are diabetic.

▶ Your baby is small (page 176).

▶ You have had runs of contractions but no cervical dilation ('false labour').

Labour may be induced if your waters have broken but contractions have not started within 24 hours (or longer depending on hospital policy).

Induction – your options

Non-medical techniques

▶ If labour is imminent, hip rolling and squatting, nipple stimulation, massage with jasmine oil, sex (or more precisely, semen) and visualization may help.

> **must know**
>
> **Is it right for you?**
> The decision to induce is not always easy. Talk with your midwife and your birth partner. Safety is, of course, the highest priority but if induction is recommended only because your due date has passed, it may be worth waiting before using medical techniques, which can be unpleasant. Up to five in every 100 babies are born more than 14 days after their due date.
>
> ▶ Double check your expected due date.
>
> ▶ If you have a five-week menstrual cycle, a 41-week pregnancy is normal.

▶ Castor oil with orange juice (60ml/2 fl oz of each) is a traditional remedy with questionable effect. It can bring on diarrhoea, and may stimulate your baby's bowels; it's not recommended if amniotic fluid volume is low, so check with your midwife.

▶ Acupuncture: treatments over few days can be very effective.

▶ A sweep: done by an experienced midwife who stretches your cervix and sweeps your membranes using her finger. It's not recommended if you have placenta praevia (page 180).

▶ Homeopathy: prescribed according to your mood and physical symptoms, often with a rapid effect.

Medical techniques

If none of the above work or if there is an urgent need for labour to begin, you will be medically induced. You and your baby will be closely monitored (see pages 126–7). If your cervix is already ripening, the effect is likely to be more rapid.

▶ Prostaglandin: inserted into your vagina every six hours to stimulate your uterus and cervix. You may feel pain for some hours before you begin to dilate and true labour begins.

▶ Oxytocin or syntocinon: a synthetic drug similar to the hormone oxytocin (see page 74) that is naturally produced by you and your baby. It is given via a drip and may bring on strong, frequent contractions. Once labour is in flow, the drip may be taken away or you may need it throughout. Artificial oxytocin may reduce natural production. If you receive artificial oxytocin, spending time with your baby, skin-to-skin, and feeding after birth helps to get the hormone flowing for both of you.

▶ Artificial rupture of the membranes (ARM): more common in a second or subsequent pregnancy, and not recommended if you have a vaginal infection such as strep B (see page 183 for more).

▶ If induction has no effect, a caesarean section may be essential.

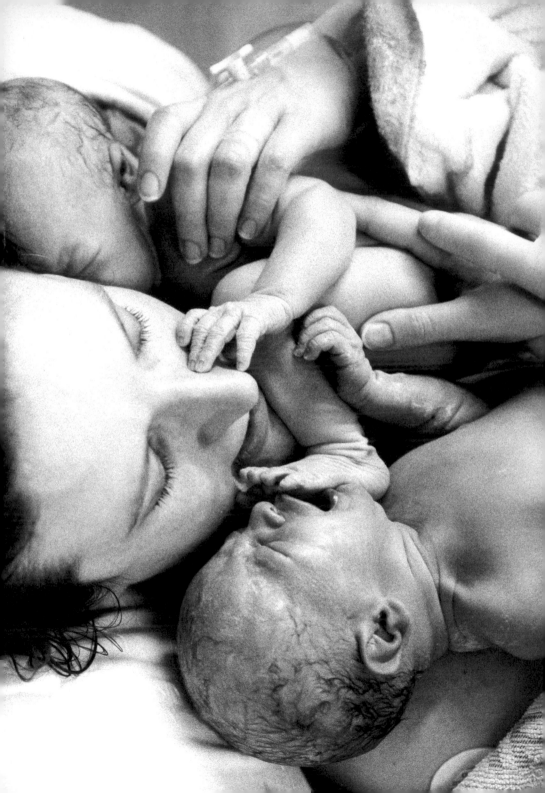

4 Labour and birth

The word 'labour' suggests hard toil. Yes, it's hard, but it is not all hard: labour may involve calm, peace, excitement and ecstatic energy as well as pain, intense difficulty and fear. It is a huge event for your baby and may be the greatest moment of your life. You will need to draw on your deepest reserves of energy, courage and determination and you will also need to let go, follow your instincts, and let the flow of labour carry you and your baby towards birth. When your baby is here, labour – and pregnancy – will seem like a lifetime ago.

'It seems as if something is emanating from this child. He seems to radiate a peace, a serenity, that he's brought from somewhere far beyond.'
Frédérick Leboyer, from *Birth without Violence*

Preparing for labour

Labour is a powerful process driven by you and your baby, fuelled by instinct and the natural forces of your body and mind. You cannot learn to give birth – but you can prepare. Preparing will help you feel more confident and, on the day, help you to stay afloat through your own journey, come what may.

must know

Breathing
Focusing on your breath brings your body and mind together in harmony: this may be one of your most powerful tools in labour.

How to prepare

In pregnancy, your body gradually loosens and your instinctive mind becomes increasingly dominant. By the time labour begins, nature has already done much of the work for you. Your preparations add to this foundation.

You will be helping yourself if you exercise regularly (pages 28–9) and you can practice some labour positions each day (pages 118–19) as you rest, read or watch television; even while you garden or peel potatoes.

Your thoughts have a huge influence over your body and your sensitivity to pain and they connect you with your baby. You can make the most of this if you choose to visualize the way you want labour to unfold, physically and emotionally (see page 91).

Arrange for someone to be with you

Research over the last 25 years has shown that having a supportive companion with you throughout labour is one of the most effective ways to enhance your experience and reduce the likelihood of complications. The effect is strongest if your support person is with you before you enter the active stage of labour. Your partner plays an important role but you may want extra (or alternative) support from a female relative or friend who has been in labour herself. Some people employ a doula or an independent midwife (see pages 42–3 and 46).

Feel your fear

Fear is a common feeling: you may fear pain, exposure, hospital or losing control; you may worry about your baby's wellbeing or that you cannot do it, or about being a parent. Most of these anxieties affect men as much as they do women and at least some fear is universal – it is natural when facing the unknown. The down side is that fear drives your reflex to flee, makes pain seem worse, blocks the flow of birthing hormones, contributes to tension and increases inhibition. The most helpful preparation may be to find your anxieties and talk about them. Some anxiety may then be less intrusive in labour and if fears arise on the day, you may find it easier to calm yourself.

Get in the know

Find out about labour and birth, your options for pain relief and your midwife's and hospital's approach. Much less tempting, but equally important to know, are some of the things that could prompt concern or intervention. You will both be in a better position to discuss your options with your birth team and to support one another.

Your baby's debut

Preparation also entails planning ahead for your baby's first experience outside the womb. Soft lights and a quiet atmosphere and the smell and feel of your skin and your loving hands are a fitting welcome. If he needs help establishing breathing, the midwives can soon pass him back to you. If you are too tired or overwhelmed to hold your baby, the hands of his father are the next best thing.

Your birth plan

Preparing a birth plan helps to focus your mind and may help you make important decisions in labour. Your plan also tells your birth team what you want – an important issue if you are cared for by a number of different people – and can include looking ahead beyond birth.

Team work

It's a good idea to create your birth plan with your partner and in consultation with your midwife or other supporters. The feeling of being in a partnership, where your wishes are known and respected, will probably increase your confidence. You can take plenty of time and can alter your plan if your views or your circumstances change. Remember that many things affect labour and it's important to have a 'plan B'. You can use the guide opposite – add or omit sections depending on your needs.

You may wish to work together to feel contractions and tune into your baby in early labour.

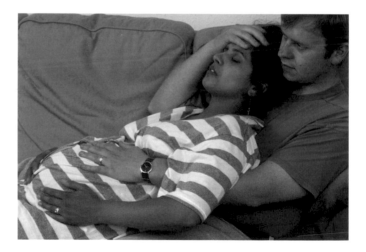

A birth plan

Labour
- I'll call my midwife when ...
- I want [name] and [name] to be with me ...
- I wish to bring things into the room (e.g. CD player, birth ball) ...
- We will prepare the following snacks and drinks ...
- My preference for monitoring is ...
- For pain relief I would like to begin with ...
- If I need further relief, my preference is ...
- I am keen/not keen to use the water pool for labour/for birth ...
- My preferences concerning being active and upright are ...
- My partner wishes to take breaks, if appropriate, every two hours ...

Birth
- My feelings about intervention are ...
- My partner is/is not keen to welcome our baby's head ...
- I wish/don't mind that the lights are dimmed and the room quiet ...
- I wish the cord to be cut after it stops pulsating/after the third stage ... by [name]
- I want to hold my baby straight away/or after he has been washed ...
- I want/don't want to try feeding in the delivery room ...
- I want/don't want oxytocin to speed up birth of the placenta ...

In the first few days
- We have asked [names] to help out at home ...
- I'd like to stay in hospital for ...
- I'd like an osteopath to visit us ...
- No visitors/lots of visitors ...

'A friend of mine talked me into deep relaxation and used hypnotherapy to guide me, telling me how the birth would go, how my body would be opening, and what would be happening to my baby. She made a CD, which I used on the day, and guided my partner so he knew what to say, how to prompt me. The birth was fantastic. People tell you that you can't prepare – but I really believe you can.'
Sarah

Signs of labour

Labour is defined as progessive cervical dilation: but your body may be actively changing for hours or days before this. One of your most pressing questions may be, 'How will I know?' Rest assured, even if you don't feel the early stages, when labour begins there's little mistaking it.

must know

Signs of early labour
If there is a sign of labour before week 37, you must call your midwife immediately. You may be advised to rest or you may need extra care to minimize the risks associated with premature birth (page 181).

Contractions

The first sign of labour may be strong contractions, but usually there is a gentle run-up with a combination of bodily changes and altered moods. You will have been having runs of Braxton-Hicks contractions for some weeks. These feel tight but are seldom painful and usually stop after an hour. Labour contractions are different because your uterus is contracting from the top down to provide the power for your baby to move down and your cervix to open. They are usually uncomfortable: you may feel aches or acute pains in your back, your uterus, your thighs, or all three, or have menstrual-type pains. Labour contractions tend to begin roughly 20 minutes apart and last for 30–45 seconds. As labour progresses, they become more closely spaced and more forceful. Ring your midwife (and go to hospital if that is your plan) when contractions are five minutes apart, or sooner if your midwife has recommended this.

Of course there are variations. You may feel intense contractions from the start, or you may experience little discomfort until your cervix is almost fully dilated. Occasionally, strong contractions last for hours or even a day or two, and then die down: this is false labour.

Breaking waters

The membranes around your baby may break before contractions begin with a flush of warm liquid or a slow flow of clear, sweet smelling fluid. Call your midwife straight away or at a sociable time: she will advise you what to do, depending on your circumstances. It's usually safe to await the onset of contractions but do avoid intercourse. Induction may be recommended if labour has not started within 24 hours (see pages 108–9).

A show

As it ripens, your cervix may release its mucus plug in a discharge, perhaps with a little blood. This can happen hours or days before labour begins and you can carry on as normal. Call your midwife immediately if you experience any bleeding.

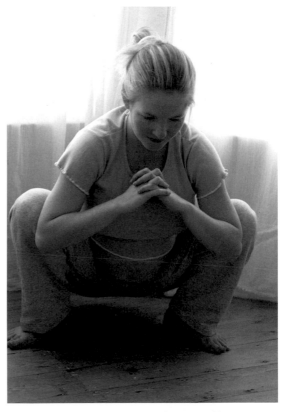

In the run-up to labour you may go into yourself as your energy is drawn to your uterus and your baby.

Other signs

The hormones that trigger labour affect every aspect of you. Your energy may change, making you 'nest' or become introspective or restless. You may have vivid dreams. Your sense of smell may also intensify and you may yearn to be in water.

Pre-labour

Some women experience changes in mood and discomfort for a few days before true labour begins. This is known as pre-labour. It's especially important to eat well and rest during this time – you'll need lots of energy in the days to come.

Positions for labour

Many images of women giving birth show them lying down. This influences the way women think they are expected to give birth, but there is unequivocal evidence that being active and upright helps labour flow and relieves pain. Your position is important for you and for your baby.

Follow your instincts

Being active does not mean that you need to be moving around constantly and it is important to rest as you maintain your energy. At times you may feel overwhelmed: that is when your partner and your midwives are there to guide you. Not all midwives are confident in supporting active birth, so it's useful to talk to your team before labour.

The positions illustrated here help your baby descend and increase the space in your pelvis and are intended as a guide – there are many variations. Practising them will make it easier on the day. For more information, see *The New Active Birth* by Janet Balaskas.

Supported squatting maximizes the space in your pelvis and helps your baby descend in the second stage. You may want support from behind or from someone in front of you.

Try to avoid lying on your back

▶ Lying on your back is the least helpful as gravity is working against the pattern of your contractions and the movement of your baby. In the second stage, lying on your back increases pressure on your perineum.

▶ When you rest, lie on your side or propped up, or kneeling with your head resting on a chair or cushion.

▶ If your baby is being constantly monitored, you will be less free to move but may still be able to adopt a supported sitting position with a pillow under your bottom.

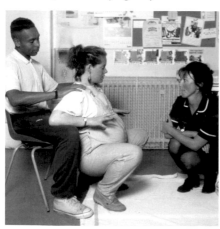

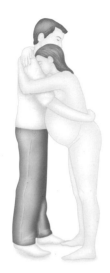

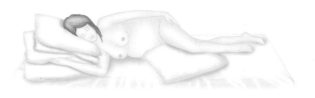

Above: Lying on your side is a restful position: a pillow between your legs will help to keep your pelvic space open. If you give birth in this position you, your midwife or partner can hold up your uppermost leg to maximize space for your baby to emerge.

Left: Walking, dancing or swaying, alone or with a partner, standing or resting against a wall, chair or bed will all support the downward force of your contractions. You can roll your hips at the same time. You may need two people to support your weight if you give birth standing: a good position for maximum opening.

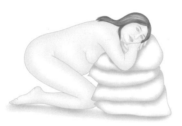

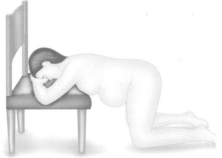

Above left and right: Kneeling with your head supported, you may rest your bottom on your heels, or raise and rotate your hips as you ride through a contraction. This is as easy in a water pool as it is on dry land. If you give birth in an all fours or kneeling position, your baby can be passed to you through your legs.

Right: Resting semi-upright is preferable to lying flat. Keep a pillow under your bottom so your perineum is slightly raised off the bed. You can sit like this in water, with a pile of towels or a blow-up pillow to raise your bottom off the base of the pool. If you give birth in this position, you may feel focused and require no assistance; or prefer another person to support you from behind.

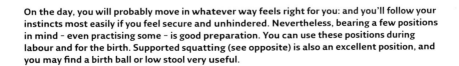

On the day, you will probably move in whatever way feels right for you: and you'll follow your instincts most easily if you feel secure and unhindered. Nevertheless, bearing a few positions in mind - even practising some - is good preparation. You can use these positions during labour and for the birth. Supported squatting (see opposite) is also an excellent position, and you may find a birth ball or low stool very useful.

Pain and pain relief in labour

Labour is painful. Ask any mother. Yet the sensations are unique: the force of labour can be powerful and invigorating even though it hurts. What's more, the pain is temporary – it does pass. Your attitude to pain, and the methods you choose for relieving it, will affect the way you feel on the day.

Natural fear, natural coping

It is completely natural to be afraid of being in pain, both in advance and when you are actually in labour. Unfortunately, fear tends to increase tension and pain, but your body is geared up for labour – ready to open, stretch and give birth, and ready to release floods of chemicals that reduce pain. Your natural ability to cope will be strongest when you feel safe and comfortable and lovingly supported, especially if the same person can stay with you throughout labour.

You may be reassured to know that nature is on your side and excited to know that there is a lot you can do to help yourself. You may also be pleased to know that medical and complementary assistance can help too: a combination may be the best option for you. Your choices depend on how labour unfolds for you and your baby.

Self-help
▶ Breathe – do not hold your breath when pain comes on; it makes it worse. As your uterus contracts, you will enhance its power if you relax.
▶ Use the space between contractions for breathing, resting, positive affirmation and focusing your energy. Drink water.
▶ Use your body: follow your urges.
▶ Hold someone's hand: contact is very powerful.
▶ Visualize – take your mind's eye into your uterus and imagine

To boost your comfort and enhance labour

May increase discomfort and/or hinder progress	What you can do
Not feeling supported	Arrange support in advance of labour
Anxiety and fear	Express your fear; draw on calming techniques
Tension	As your uterus contracts, you need to relax – your uterus is able to provide lots of power; breathe
Dehydration	Have water and ice cubes to hand, and a water spray for your face
Low blood sugar	Prepare slow-burning snacks (pages 20–3) to eat, if you can hold them down
Posture	You can get upright and active if you have the energy and others can support you
Being too cold or too hot	Your birth partner can help to regulate temperature
Feeling out of control	Express yourself, use support of your companions, try homeopathy Nux Vomica
Feeling embarrassed	Ask to be covered; ask for the person who makes you feel nervous to leave the room; remember that whatever you are doing is your natural way of coping; try homeopathic Natrum Mur
Pain	Use calming techniques, massage and visualization; consider medical pain relief
Bright lights and noise	Dim the lights, ask for quiet
Different or unwelcome people in the room	Your birth partner may be able to minimize disruption where possible
Awkward positioning	If your baby's position is problematic, intervention may be needed

the walls expanding, your baby descending, and your cervix opening. Imagine blood, energy and natural pain-relieving endorphins flowing freely.

▶ Try water – you may want to get in the birth pool.

Birth partner tips

▶ Guide her breathing, talk her into relaxation and a visualization perhaps.

▶ Reassure her and assist communication with the midwives/doctors.

▶ Support her physically so she can be comfortable.

- Remind her of her affirmations.
- Give her drinks, cool her brow with a wet flannel, take charge of any music she wants.
- Apply complementary techniques, such as massage, aromatherapy, acupressure, homeopathy.
- Look after yourself: eat and drink to keep your energy up.
- Try not to take any outbursts or criticisms personally.
- You may need to step aside or leave the room if you are increasing her anxiety; or if you need a break.

Water

The soothing effect of being immersed in body-temperature water helps to reduce muscle tension and stimulates hormones that relieve pain and help you feel positive. Water can also increase the ease with which your vagina opens. If you are comfortable, feel well supported and have no complications, you may want to give birth in the pool. Water babies often seem especially contented and peaceful.

Safety in water

Birthing pools in hospitals are carefully kept at an optimum temperature and are sterilized before use. If you rent a pool to use at home, try it out before labour: practise moving, getting comfortable and stabilizing the temperature. Sterilize it before labour. For more information, see www.waterbirth.co.uk.

If your baby is born in the water, he has a strong 'dive reflex' that prevents him from taking a breath until there's contact with cooler air.

You'll feel safer if you feel comfortable: you can use blow-up pillows and rubber rings, a plastic stool or chair or rolled-up towels and you can take many different positions.

When to use the pool

It is best to reserve the pool until you have passed 6cm dilation. Earlier than this, the relaxing effect may slow your progress. You may use the pool for birth and/or after birth, when you will probably all feel blissfully relaxed.

When not to use the pool

▶ If you don't feel drawn to it – even if it was your plan. Leave at any time if you don't feel comfortable.

▶ If there are signs of foetal distress; your baby may need closer monitoring and/or assistance.

▶ If you want an epidural.

▶ If labour is progressing slowly in the first stage, or, in the second stage, if you feel you will have more power to push on dry land.

Midwife-led pain relief

In addition to natural methods and emotional reasurrance, midwives offer a range of pain relief. Your midwife may help you re-inhabit your body and, no longer distracted and distressed by pain, feel in control and able to deal with your contractions.

Gas and air or 'entonox' (inhaling nitrous oxide)

This takes the edge off the pain within a minute of inhalation and may make you feel light-headed (it's also called laughing gas). It's quite highly rated. The gas may make you thirsty, dizzy and vague; and you may be less inclined to follow your instincts to change position. It doesn't seem to reduce efficiency of contractions. The effects on a baby are unknown.

Intradermal water injections or intracutaneous sterile water blocks

Sterile-water injections, also known as sterile-water papules (swp) are relatively new in the UK. Placed precisely at points on your lower back, they can bring incredible relief from lower back pain, although they won't reduce abdominal pain. They give relief within minutes, lasting for up to two hours. There are no known side effects for mother or baby, although the injections themselves do sting.

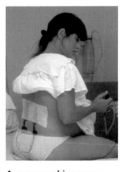

A TENS machine uses electrical impulses, via the skin on your back, to alter the transmission of pain signals to your brain. Many women use TENS early in labour. Later on its value falls. It gives a good sense of being in control and has no apparent side effects. You can hire a unit from your hospital, midwife or pharmacy.

Local anaesthetic

You'll need this if you have torn during birth and require stitching. Your midwife will inject it into your perineum: this gives a slight sting then you feel nothing so you can focus on your baby (and your tea and toast).

Opioids and tranquillizers

Pethidine is the most commonly used opioid, administered by injection and with anti-nausea medication. It's not highly rated. Although it dulls the pain, kicks in quickly and may allow you to sleep for a bit, it can bring on wooziness, nausea, dizziness and even hallucination and make labour seem unreal. These effects do pass though. There is little research into side effects but a link is acknowledged with an affect on a baby's heartbeat and an increase in the likelihood of breathing difficulties and reduced alertness after birth. This is more likely if the drug is used close to birth.

Tranquillizers are less commonly used to induce sleep, usually in early labour. Considerations and side effects are similar to opioids.

Consultant-led care

This is only available in a consultant-led unit. If self-help measures and midwife-administered relief are not sufficient, or you require powerful relief urgently, a consultant anaesthetist (sometimes together with an obstetrician) will come to give you anaesthetic relief.

Epidural

An epidural has become something of a golden ticket; many women praise it for completely taking the pain away and helping them to be mentally and

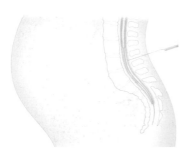

emotionally present and enjoy the birth. It has other benefits, too, including reducing high blood pressure and, for some, assisting cervical dilation. A mobile epidural is preferable; a full epidural may leave you paralysed from the waist down.

An epidural involves the insertion of a fine tube into the epidural space in your spine, through which anaesthetic is administered. In most cases it relieves lower back and abdominal pain within 10-20 minutes. You can use it for a short period then give birth without it; or you can have the anaesthetic topped up for the remainder of your labour. You'll need to give your permission, and will have a drip in your arm to help keep your blood pressure stable.

Although the incidence of side effects is low, there can be disadvantages to an epidural. Pain relief may not be complete, and having an epidural does raise the likelihood that you will need intervention. Your blood pressure may drop, making you feel faint (usually temporarily); contractions often lose power and it is more difficult to bear down; there is an increased risk of foetal distress. After birth, there is a risk of pain in your back, shoulders, neck or head continuing for hours and, less commonly, days.

Pudendal block

The pudendal nerves in your vagina can be blocked to relieve pain, usually in conjunction with a forceps or ventouse delivery. An obstetrician can give this without an anaesthetist present.

Spinal block

This anaesthetic is typically reserved for an emergency caesarean if an epidural is not already in place. It gives relief for 4-6 hours but there's a higher chance of having a headache afterwards.

> **watch out!**
>
> **Extreme pain**
> Extreme pain may signal an underlying problem, such as awkward positioning of your baby: a midwife is trained to interpret these signs and detect problems.

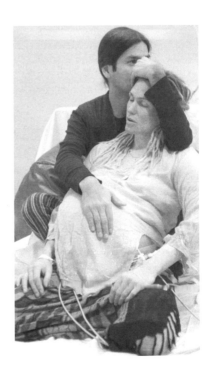

Monitoring in labour

Your midwife is your guardian: she is here to keep an eye on you and your baby and will be alert to any signs of complications. There are a number of ways to monitor you both. They include assessing your mood and state of mind, observing the power and spacing of your contractions, and monitoring your baby's heartbeat.

Foetal heart monitoring

Monitoring a baby's heart rate in labour has been a widespread practice since the 1970s. A baby's heart rate slows at the start of a contraction and rises at the end. If it is unusually rapid, this may signal stress, pain or fear. A slow beat may signal a reduction in oxygen and is cause for concern since prolonged oxygen deprivation may cause damage to one or more areas of the brain.

What if the reading is low?

Changing position or becoming upright may help to normalize your baby's heartbeat by improving circulation and blood supply to the placenta. If you have been given syntocinon, the dose may be reduced.

Short-term deceleration is usually not a cause for concern: babies draw on stores of glucose energy if oxygen supply falls. Long-term deceleration does carry a risk and birth may need to be speeded up: either with forceps or ventouse, or with a caesarean.

Hand-held monitors

Hand-held monitors can be used in many positions. They cannot be used for continuous monitoring:

▶ The fetoscope is like a stethoscope and lets your midwife hear your baby's heartbeat by placing the stethoscope's bell end on your abdomen.

▶ The 'doptone' or sonic aid uses ultrasound to pick up a baby's heartbeat and can be used in water.

Cardiotocograph (CTG)
CTG is a monitor fixed to your abdomen with a belt. It uses ultrasound to register your contractions and your baby's heartbeat. CTG can be used while you are sitting, lying, kneeling or squatting, but is more awkward than a hand-held monitor. You may have CTG monitoring for 20–30 minutes when you are admitted to hospital, and perhaps again at a later stage. Constant CTG monitoring is often recommended if you receive medication to augment contractions (such as syntocinon); if you have an epidural; if there are concerns about your baby; or if you have a 'high-risk' pregnancy.

Internal monitoring
Less commonly, a baby is monitored through an electrode placed on his scalp, via the mother's cervix. A blood sample may be taken from the scalp to measure blood-oxygen levels.

Monitoring: pros and cons
Opinions about monitoring vary, with some people praising its value, and others bemoaning its interference and inaccuracy. As an alert to potential problems it may save lives even though some readings may not be accurate. Routine monitoring for prolonged periods (e.g. for 10–30 minutes every two to four hours in the first stage) may disturb the natural rhythm of labour and impede progress, and this could increase the need for assistance. There is also an issue of false readings, which may make a mother afraid. Evidence to date suggests that routine continuous foetal monitoring does not improve outcomes. You may wish to specify a preference for intermittent monitoring unless there is concern for your baby. For a discussion on monitoring, see www.birthingnaturally.net.

Stage one: opening your cervix

The first stage of labour is triggered by a symphony of hormones released by you, by your baby and by the placenta. They act on your cervix and uterus, awaken your birthing power, and they support your baby. As the symphony crescendos, you and your baby enter the transition stage that precedes birth.

The latent and active phases

Although in practice labour tends to flow seamlessly, different phases have been defined. The 'latent phase', when your cervix dilates from 0–3cm, lasts from two to 12 hours. It usually begins with mild contractions, but this varies – you might be unaware that labour has begun, or you might feel continual pain.

The 'active phase' begins when your cervix dilates beyond 3cm and it may last for up to eight hours. You can expect contractions to get increasingly intense and more frequent.

Contractions

Take one contraction at a time as tightening wells up and then passes. Let go of thoughts about what others are doing around you, and what is to come. Do what feels comfortable as you ride through each swell. Most importantly, breathe. Breathe into and through the pain: holding your breath will increase discomfort and reduce your energy. Your birth partner

The first stage	
Your cervix dilates from 0 to 10cm	
Time taken	2–20 hours
Pain relief options	Breathing, movement and hip rolls, water, massage, gas and air, epidural
Energy conservation	Regular healthy snacks; resting if contractions are mild
Most difficult part	Transition

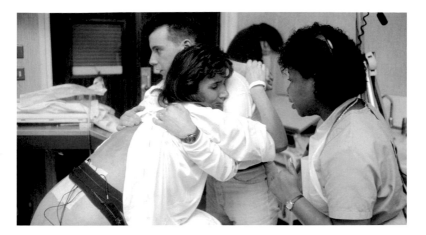

can help you focus and you might find it helps to visualize your cervix opening and your baby pushing downwards (see page 91).

Transition (5 minutes to 2 hours)

When your cervix has dilated to 10cm, contractions change quality, duration and frequency and you may enter an altered state. Hormones quieten the logical, thinking part of your brain and your instincts come to the fore. You may roar like a lioness; you may be in a silent trance; you may moan and move your body in a wave-like rhythm. Your own 'birth song' is an expression of your birthing power.

At the end of transition, fear is extremely common: it's a good sign, fuelled by a rush of adrenalin that also acts on your uterus to stimulate your reflex to bear down and give birth. Even fear of death can be part of the flow of labour. Express any fear you feel; holding it in may prolong this stage. Soon your mood will change.

'There is a fear of labour being an emergency. It's not – you take your time, you let your body do the work, you feel, you go into yourself, you go into your dark room. There will be stages when you don't feel you can go on. When that happens, you are nearly there.'
Sari, doula and mother

To push or not to push?

At the end of transition most women feel a surge of energy and a consuming urge to bear down. These are signs that cervical dilation is complete and your baby is ready to pass through your cervix and descend your birth canal.

Occasionally, the urge comes before full dilation: but pushing too soon may cause your cervix to swell and hinder your baby's descent. Your midwife may check your cervix. If the time isn't right, try kneeling with your head on a cushion with your bottom in the air: this releases the pressure from your baby's head.

Slow progress?

Every hospital and midwife has different guidelines for what's considered an excessive time during each stage. The timings mark a point where you or your baby may need help to move on. Timings are not usually rigid but knowing your hospital's/midwife's policy in advance will help you know what to expect, should your progress be slow on the day.

If you travel to hospital or change location, your contractions may lose intensity. As you settle into the new space and begin to relax, labour may pick up:

▶ The homeopathic remedy Pulsatilla can help.
▶ Jasmine or clarysage essential oils may help.

Several other factors may cause slow cervical dilation, including your tiredness and state of mind, and your sensitivity to pain. If you have been lying down, you could try moving or altering your position: this may gradually boost your contractions. With the guidance and help of your partner or other supporters you may be able to overcome some of these – see the table on page 121. Your baby's position and size is also relevant.

Assisting labour
Complementary care

If you have the knowledge or a professional is with you, using complementary care such as aromatherapy, acupuncture or homeopathy may give you the boost you need. Being in water may help to release tension; you could try this late in the first stage.

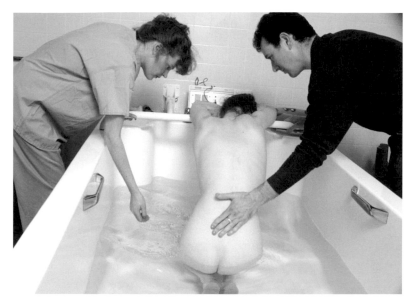

Many women are drawn to water during labour, for security and comfort.

Breaking your waters (amniotomy or ARM)

Your midwife may recommend this if your contractions are weak or uncoordinated and you are nearing full dilation. In skilled hands this can be done quickly, although you may feel slight discomfort. Artificial rupture of the membranes (ARM) is usually followed by much stronger contractions. If contractions don't pick up after ARM, you may need further assistance (oxytocin/caesarean).

Augmentation with oxytocin

Delivering synthetic oxytocin (syntocinon) via a drip increases the power of contractions. Some women feel encouraged and more in control; others are shocked by a rapid increase in pain and request an epidural and/or further assistance. Oxytocin may be linked with distress for some babies. If you have had a previous caesarean or other abdominal surgery augmentation is better avoided or done with care.

If attempts at enhancing progress don't work, or your baby is in distress, a caesarean section or other intervention may be needed (see pages 138–45).

Stage two: your baby is born

Once your cervix has fully dilated, your baby is able to pass into your vagina. As your baby moves downwards and your contractions take on a new quality, you will feel yourself bearing down or pushing. You are on the threshold of birth.

The power of birth

Many women enter a completely altered state of consciousness now. You may feel downward pressure, forceful contractions and pain so strongly that you surrender to your body and your baby, and have little need to focus on actively pushing. If you need to harness more power to bear down, using an upright position will help. It will also encourage your baby's descent and increase the space in your pelvis. It may feel good to kneel with your head and hands resting on a chair and someone helping you.

It's common to have a burst of energy following transition, but if the second stage is long, your energy may dip. Your birth partner can help you use techniques to rest well between contractions and harness your energy as you need it.

You may cry out, 'I can't do it, I can't.' Usually the refrain is, 'Yes you can, you are doing it.' Your midwife will be watching you closely and will continue to monitor your baby's heartbeat. She will focus on your vagina for the first sign of your baby's head as it crowns.

You may feel stinging and incredible force and volume – as if your whole lower body is descending. You may be afraid, and it's natural to have a surge of adrenalin. Some birth practitioners believe fear triggers a 'foetal ejection reflex'. Feel the fear: be with it, it is normal, it will pass. Let go of any worries that you may defecate: if this happens you will not notice and your midwife will clear it away.

Birth

Once your baby's head has crowned, your midwife may gently guide you to avoid pushing too hard; letting your baby descend and gradually opening is gentler for you both. Your midwife may help by inserting a finger between your baby's head and your vaginal lips (or it may be necessary to use further intervention with forceps or ventouse – see page 139). First his head will be born then, after another one or two contractions, his body.

Few words can adequately describe the emotional and physical mixture of pain, pleasure, awe, relief and power that accompany birth. Everyone in the room will be moved, even professionals who have been at hundreds of births. Your baby is here.

The first breath

Your baby will instinctively take a breath as he makes contact with the air (or once he has surfaced from the water in the pool) and feels the contact of hands on his body. If this doesn't happen, your midwife will clear his nose and mouth with gentle suction and, when she is happy that your baby is breathing effectively, pass him to you. Some babies need a little more help to establish regular breathing at a 'resuscitaire' before being reunited with their mums.

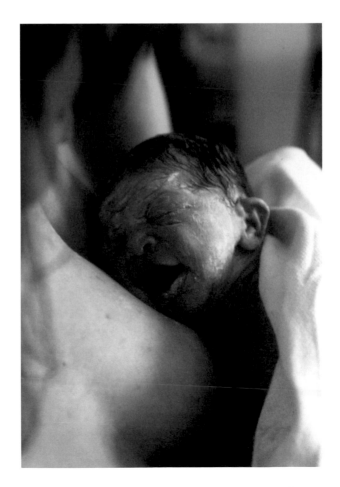

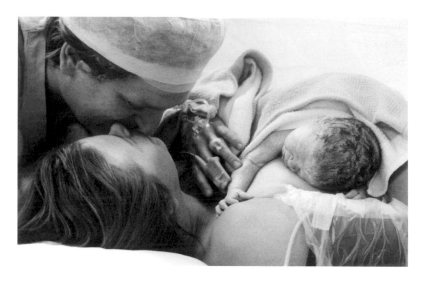

First contact

Providing all has gone well, when your midwife or your partner passes your baby to you, the best thing for him is to lie him on your stomach or chest, his skin against yours. You can lay your hands over his back and a light blanket will keep you both warm. As he rests with his legs and arms tucked in, he will smell your familiar smell and hear your heartbeat. Your baby will be able to uncurl in his own time and you may leave the cord in place if you do not wish to cut it straight away. If you are not feeling up to it, your partner may want to hold your baby: skin to skin if possible. There is nothing like it.

'It was just perfect, when she popped out I had her head in my left hand and her body in my right. It was absolutely wonderful, experiencing that whole journey like I was with her for the whole thing. I am so proud of Jenny, so proud of her, she was brilliant. A cold flannel was all the anaesthetic she needed. It didn't take her long to become a wolf, low moaning, she was fantastic. I'm so happy.'
Mike

Your baby's arrival

Some babies arrive with gusto and great energy, instantly cry and soon stretch their arms and legs out, eyes wide as they look around. Some are quiet and calm. Some suckle and feed within minutes of birth. Others rest and relax as they orientate themselves and greet their parents. The range of post-birth feelings is no different from what mothers experience.

If you need help

If you are exhausted or there is concern for you or for your baby, you may need some extra help. This could range from an oxytocin drip to boost the power of your contractions, to assistance with ventouse. Find out more on pages 138–41.

Cutting the cord

The cord delivers oxygen to your baby from the placenta while he establishes normal breathing. Then, as your baby's lungs expand, changes in placental oxygen levels close the umbilical artery, and blood flow through the cord stops. The cord becomes pale and still, and is no longer providing oxygen. The most natural approach, providing there are no complications, is to allow the cord to stop pulsating before clamping and cutting it. If you feel well after the birth and wish to hold your baby, the cord can be cut after the placenta is born. More and more dads are now choosing to cut the cord and this remains an option after a caesarean.

Clamping the cord within seconds of birth may result in some blood being trapped in the placenta. As a result, less remains in your baby's circulation, and this is thought to increase the likelihood of needing extra oxygen. If the cord is wound tightly around your baby's neck or resuscitation is needed, then the cord will be cut so that your baby can be taken to the resuscitaire.

Some hospitals routinely inject synthetic oxytocin to speed up delivery of the placenta; if you are given this, the cord needs to be cut so your baby does not receive the drug.

> **must know**
>
> **Your baby's APGAR test**
> One minute after birth, and again at five minutes, your midwife assesses your baby. The results indicate your baby's wellbeing: seven or above (out of a total of ten), and she is doing well. Five or below, and some extra assistance may be needed (usually some help with breathing). Babies who score low in the first test usually score higher five minutes later.
> A Appearance
> P Pulse
> G Grimace/cry
> A Activity
> R Respiration (breathing)

Stage three: greeting your baby and placenta

As you rest with your baby, you enter the third stage of labour. You make eye contact and smell your baby for the first time, looking at his face and his tiny lips as they stretch and pout. The birth of the placenta is imminent: usually, it's simple.

Hello, baby

If you are feeling strong enough to hold your baby while you sit propped up, you may be unable to resist the compulsion to touch him – with your hands, your lips, perhaps your cheek – and to look into his eyes. You may instinctively massage him with a rhythm that matches the rhythm of contractions of your heart, and this will feel familiar and calming.

This is as nature intends: you are getting to know one another. And, inside your brain, this first contact of eyes and skin triggers more production of the hormone oxytocin. Not only does this make you and your baby feel loved up, it also helps you relax and it triggers further contractions, which will help your placenta to emerge.

If you wish to feed your baby, and he is ready and suckles with ease, this will further boost your oxytocin levels. But it is by no means essential: not all babies or mothers want to start feeding immediately.

How does it feel?

The contractions in this last stage will not be as severe as before (but they tend to be stronger with each successive birth). The placenta is usually born within 30 minutes, with a final, gentle push. Your midwife may gently massage your abdomen to help. There is no sensation of stretching; rather there is a soft, warm feeling. If you wish to see and feel the amazing organ that has been sustaining your baby, note it in your birth plan.

After labour

Once your placenta is born, your midwife will examine you and stitch you, if this is needed. She will measure your baby's length and head circumference and weigh him. If you wish your baby to be washed, your midwife can do this – your baby will have traces of blood on his skin and will need to be gently cleaned if he has passed a motion. Beneath this superficial covering, your baby will be coated in the white vernix that has moisturized him in the womb. It is preferable not to wash this off because it protects him: instead you can gently massage it into his skin over the coming days.

The next stage is for rest. You may want to take a bath on your own or with your baby and partner, or settle into bed. If your baby is sleeping, you can sleep too: you both need the rest.

Assisting the birth of the placenta

▶ The birth of the placenta is a natural part of labour. Sometimes, it may be delayed or there may be excessive blood loss.

▶ Some hospitals routinely give synthetic oxytocin or syntometrine to speed up the birth and reduce these risks; or offer the injection if the placenta is not born within 30 or 60 minutes. If an injection is given, the cord will be clamped immediately before and your placenta will be born within five minutes.

▶ You can discuss your preferences for this stage as part of your birth plan.

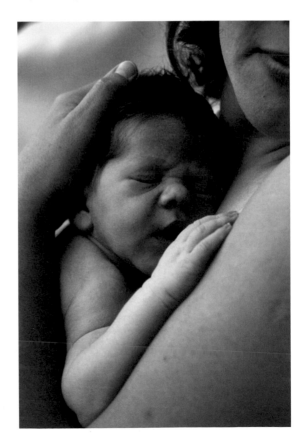

Extra help for labour and birth

Labour is not entirely in your control, nor in the midwives'; it is a dynamic process involving you and your baby and is influenced by your bodies, your emotions, your environment and the people with you. You can take measures to reduce the likelihood that you will need assistance, but you cannot take out any guarantee.

good to know

Help yourself
You may want to use the preparation advice (page 103) and consider factors that hinder progress (page 121).

Normal, natural and assisted birth

▶ A 'normal' birth is vaginal birth without intervention; even if this follows medical assistance (e.g. with oxytocin), pain relief or complementary care.

▶ A 'natural' birth is one where labour progresses without medical assistance or pain relief is used, and a baby is born vaginally.

▶ An 'assisted' birth is one where a baby needs physical help to be born; with forceps, ventouse or caesarean. An episiotomy provides assistance but not intervention if your baby is born without further intervention.

Why might intervention be needed?

The two most likely factors that prompt intervention are difficulty in the second stage and your baby's distress. Behind these lie a number of possible factors.

▶ **Your experience at the time:** how you feel, the strength and regularity of contractions, your environment and other people in your space. Other influences include confidence, position, hydration, comfort and energy levels.

▶ **Your baby's position and fit in your pelvis:** he may be lying in an awkward position (pages 105–7) or may be large relative to your pelvis. If your baby's head does not rotate in labour, this may have an impact (more common with an epidural).

► **Foetal distress:** If your baby's heart rate indicates distress, it may be safest for your baby for birth to be speeded up.

► **Your condition:** A number of 'high-risk' conditions precipitate intervention.

► **Pain relief:** Some methods of pain relief may decrease the efficiency of your contractions and reduce your focus and stamina (pages 124–5).

Assisting birth

Episiotomy

An episiotomy is a cut that widens your vaginal opening. It is done after a local anaesthetic, usually to hasten the moment of birth once your baby's head has crowned. You may need to have your legs in stirrups during the procedure and for the birth. If your back is slightly raised and supported, this will work in your favour. After the birth of the placenta, the episiotomy cut will be stitched (this takes 20–30 minutes) and you may be able to hold your baby if you wish. Your vagina will feel tender and bruised while it heals (see also page 185).

Ventouse

A ventouse is a plastic or metal suction cup. The cup is carefully placed on your baby's head and, as you push with a contraction, it is gently pulled. You may not need an episiotomy and may not tear. Some midwives are trained to use ventouse, but it is currently more common for an obstetrician to be called. After a ventouse delivery, your baby's head may appear swollen: swelling resulting from suction pressure settles in a few days.

Forceps

Forceps may be recommended if your baby's head is in your vaginal canal and birth needs to be speeded up or he appears to be stuck. The instrument is like a pair of spoons. Following an episiotomy to widen your vaginal opening, the forceps are eased

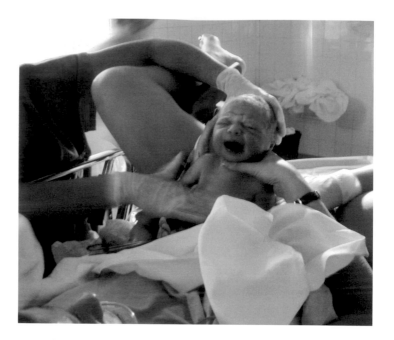

around your baby's head. As you push with a contraction, your obstetrician will gently pull. Your midwife will guide you, and will help you push with your contractions if you have had an epidural and cannot feel them. She may also assist the obstetrician. After a forceps delivery, your baby may have marks on his head and cheeks. Some forceps babies have head pain for hours or days: a headache is most effectively soothed with frequent feeding and loving touch. Osteopathy will also help to relieve trauma and you may both use homeopathy, such as Arnica, to help the bruising heal.

How might you feel after intervention?

Revisiting your birth experience is part of the transition into parenthood. It's an important aspect of your emotional adjustment and, for a woman, is part of postnatal healing. Sometimes the emotional impact of birth does not become apparent until weeks or months after the event.

You may be relieved that your baby has arrived safely and accept all that happened. Alternatively, you may be shocked or upset. You may have felt emotionally absent during the birth and feel disorientated. A lot depends on the situation that led to intervention and how you were cared for. Your personal expectations contribute to your feelings and both women and men can feel as if they have failed or been 'not good enough'. Talking about what happened and how you feel is normal and helpful – to your partner, friends, midwife or doctor. If you are angry about the way things were handled by your medical team, it's important to discuss the situation. If you feel very shaken up, unhappy or 'spaced out', consider talking to a midwife counsellor (who may be on the staff at the hospital). This could bring relief from uncomfortable and confusing feelings.

How might your baby feel?

Every baby is unique. Some seem vibrant and relaxed after what seemed to be a traumatic delivery, while others appear shocked or dazed. Your baby's reaction reflects not only the nature of his birth – but also his personality, what he has experienced in pregnancy and his physical health.

Loving contact is vital, and frequent feeding will soothe him; the sucking action also helps to relieve pressure pains in his head. Osteopathy and massage are believed to help to relieve pain and emotional trauma. You too have healing hands. Let your finger tips lightly touch your baby's head and allow them to find their way around his body and stroke out any trauma, inviting balance. If you are worried about your baby at any time, ask a midwife to check him or request a paediatric check.

In the long term, your baby will adapt most easily if he is welcomed and his needs are met. The experience of birth, many behavioural scientists believe, is significant in how a person experiences life – difficult, a struggle, easy or painful. If a baby is traumatized, loving care can help to bring early resolution.

Caesarean birth

As many as one in four women give birth by caesarean in parts of the UK. If you are advised to have a caesarean (also called a c-section), knowing the basics will help you look forward to birth, welcome your baby and recover afterwards.

Elective caesarean

A caesarean may be planned in advance for reasons that make it the safest option for both you and your baby. Sometimes the operation is essential (e.g. with placenta praevia – see page 180) and sometimes it is optional (e.g. with twins). Your obstetricians

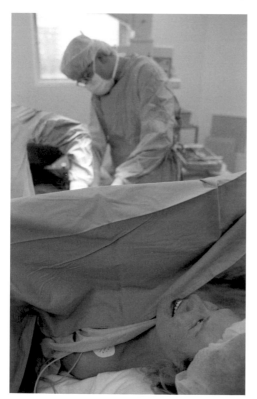

may support your choice if you want a c-section for emotional reasons (e.g. you have had a previous traumatic birth).

Emergency caesarean

When there is concern about your baby before labour begins spontaneously and your baby needs to be born urgently, or your team feels that a caesarean is the safest way forward once labour has begun, this is an emergency caesarean. Your experience will reflect the attitude of your doctors and midwives and the extent to which you feel informed. You may be nervous but relieved; or upset and frightened. If you need to be transferred, either from home to hospital, or from a low-risk unit to a larger centre, the upheaval and the waiting can be nerve racking. Your birth partner is there for you, and you may draw on the relaxation and breathing exercises you have practised.

The procedure

A c-section is carried out in the operating theatre in the care of a team including a midwife and anaesthetist and a registrar, senior registrar or consultant obstetrician. A paediatrician may also be present. Your partner will probably be welcome to stay, if he wishes to.

You will be asked to sign a consent form, given support tights to reduce the risk of blood clotting, and a urinary catheter will be fitted. This is removed around 24 hours later. If you already have an epidural in place, this can be topped up; alternatively you may be given a spinal block (see page 125). Only in an acute emergency is a general anaesthetic preferable.

In experienced hands, and providing there are no unforeseen complications, your abdomen can be opened and your baby born within 10–15 minutes. Carefully stitching the wound takes up to 30 minutes; during this time your partner may hold your baby beside you.

Emotions of a caesarean

After a c-section, most women are delighted to meet their baby and to have avoided potential problems, or to have left a difficult labour behind them. Some women, though, feel they have failed. If you are upset, it is important to talk about your feelings and you may need to spend time going over the experience with a midwife, anaesthetist or doctor.

watch out!

Infected wound
If your wound
becomes red or
feels tender, let
your midwife
know: it may
signal an
infection.

Afterwards with your baby

You may hold your baby in the recovery room or wait until you are back in the ward. Your partner and midwives can help you get comfortable. Successful feeding is just as likely as after a vaginal birth.

You will not be able to bend and pick up your baby or bathe her for several days; others can do this for you. But you can hold her. If your partner is on hand, holding and nappy changes present a great opportunity for bonding to begin. At home you need to take it easy: follow the advice of your hospital and arrange to have people around who can help for several weeks.

Recovery

The pain in your wound will be greatest in the first few days; you can top up your epidural or you may be given injections or suppositories. Some people are virtually pain free in a few days but discomfort can persist for several weeks.

Begin to move around as soon as you feel well enough, but take care not to overdo it. Walking helps to realign your muscles and improve circulation. Don't forget to wear support tights: the risk of thrombosis is greatest one week after birth. Consider homeopathy, such as Arnica or Staphysagria, to improve healing, and osteopathy (see page 47) for your baby, particularly if the operation was an emergency.

You can begin gentle yoga (see page 30) and postnatal exercises within four days, but you need to abstain from aerobic exercise for ten weeks.

The next pregnancy: another caesarean?

If the reason that led to one caesarean is not present in the next pregnancy, you may aim for a vaginal birth: 60–80% of women who have had a caesarean give birth vaginally the second time round.

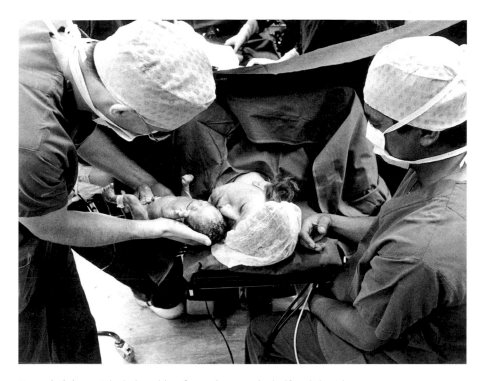

'I was in labour, I'd tried pushing for an hour and a half and they'd tried forceps. The doctors weren't reassuring or informative, in fact some were just horrid. Then they said things aren't happening, we ought to give you a c-section. I felt relieved that it was being taken out of my hands and that it wasn't that I wasn't doing enough. As it was, she was round the wrong way. The anaesthetist was fantastic, not with medical info but by talking to us and keeping us calm.

'I couldn't bear to try a normal labour again. I've had two more caesareans since, and both were fine. If you're told you need a caesarean, don't be afraid – it is OK: for my part my pelvic floor has never been so good! The big thing is, they will give you as much pain relief as you want. Afterwards it's good to be grounded – you recover more quickly and have more time with your baby. A positive rather than a negative.'

Becca

After birth: you and your baby

You may be so moved when you hold your baby that you feel as if you are in a new world, and everything is perfect. Alternatively, you may be surprised that things are not as you expected. Babies are no more uniform than adults, and there is a huge variation of 'normal' appearance and behaviour.

Is this normal?

You have seen pictures of smooth-skinned cherubs but yours is red and spotty. And other mums look radiant but you feel knackered and sore. Your baby is howling but the one in the next room seldom stirs. Don't worry. These, like a multitude of variations, are normal. Some things will change within hours or days as the hormones from pregnancy and birth alter and you and your baby adapt to what has just happened.

Your real baby
These are normal:
▶ Spots
▶ Red complexion
▶ Yellowy skin
▶ Swollen breast tissue
▶ For girls, some bleeding from the vagina
▶ Wrinkled skin (it's been wet for nine months)
▶ Sneezing and sniffing (he needs to clear his airways)
▶ Black poo within 48 hours of birth; with yellow-brown runny poo to follow; greenish if you bottle feed
▶ Crying without tears
▶ A reaction to noise or quick movements with arms and legs outstretched like a star fish (this is what is known as the startle reflex).

After the birth: what happens to you

▶ You will pass blood after the birth – for anything from five days to eight or nine weeks (even if you have had a caesarean). The flow varies from woman to woman. Use pads, not tampons, and consider disposable pants while your flow is heavy – if you've had a c-section, they go over your scar so they don't rub.

▶ Your breasts will feel swollen and may be sore.

▶ Your nipples will tingle in response to your baby's presence and cry.

▶ You may feel bruised around your vagina.

▶ Your vagina may sting when you pass urine – particularly if you have been grazed or have had stitches.

▶ You may feel nervous about pooing – the fear is always greater than the reality.

▶ You will be physically tired.

▶ You will be thirsty – drink plenty of water.

▶ You may be elated or have a sense of anticlimax – both are normal.

▶ You will feel tightenings in your abdomen as your uterus begins to contract. The sensation may be painful, particularly when you are breastfeeding.

---

watch out!

Concerning signs for your baby
If you notice any of the following, ask a member of the ward staff or your health visitor for advice:
Any difficulty breathing, e.g. fast, shallow, grunting.
Floppiness.
Rigidity.
A high-pitched cry.
No startle reaction to loud noise or sudden movement.
If your baby feels very hot or very cold.
If your baby does not wet her nappy for four hours or more.
If your baby does not pass a motion within 72 hours.
If your baby is not interested in feeding.

Signs that you need extra attention
If you feel faint.
If you pass blood clots.
If you are exhausted and pale three days or more after birth (could be a sign of anaemia).
If you have swollen calves.
If you have bad head or back pain.
If you have sharp or continual abdominal pain (a possible sign of infection).

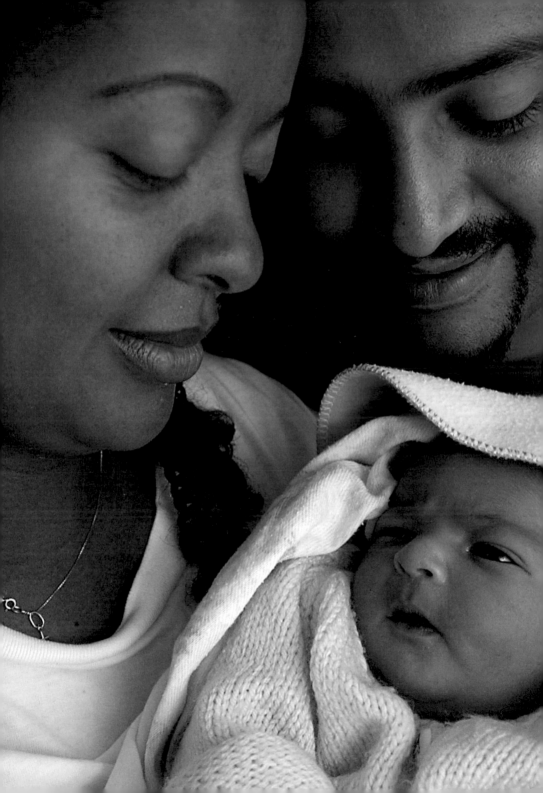

5 The early days

The birth is over and your baby is here: nine months of waiting and life begins anew. Your baby still feels as if you and she are one. The sensation of being separated from other people is completely alien, but being held and feeling the familiar rise and fall of your breath and the rhythm of your walk and your heartbeat gives her comfort and security. A mother's embrace is best; a father's a close second. From this safe space she will entice you to fall in love with her and awaken your instinctual ability to respond to her needs.

'You do not have to be perfect. You just need to be open and willing to listen to your baby and learn what she needs. By loving and trusting yourself and your baby, you will be doing wonderfully well. You will soon discover you know far more than you realise about how to be with your baby. Trust your intuition, and parent from your heart not your head. Enjoy. '
Kitty Hagenbach, mother and psychotherapist

Settling in

Often, the days after birth have a magical, soft-focus quality. You may enjoy a 'babymoon', either alone with the phone unplugged and a 'do not disturb' sign on the door, or with your family and friends around to take care of practical tasks.

Dancing together

Unconsciously, babies and parents dance together, drawing one another into intimacy and mirroring each other's facial expressions and moods, heartbeats and breathing patterns. The dance of first encounter is curious and gentle. You may find it comforting, for it is so natural, as well as frightening, for it is so new.

Baby, baby

Your baby is unlike any other in the world: an individual with a matchless genetic pattern and a unique life story. But like every other, she is driven to communicate and to form relationships. She knows who you are from your smell, your heartbeat and your voice and will let you know how she's feeling with her eyes, body movements and with small noises and louder crying. You may see her smile (despite the myths that it can't happen so early). She's a fast learner too. Within hours she will try to copy you and within days she can distinguish your face from every other.

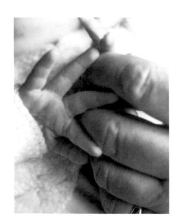

Mirror, mirror

You and your baby mirror one another. You'll unconsciously mimic her mouth movements, for instance, and she yours. Just watch – every adult does the same when caught in the gaze of a new baby. You also mirror one another emotionally.

Mirroring helps you to bond, but your baby also needs to see her reflection in you to learn about life: about language, feelings, communication, and being part of a family. You may also learn about yourself from watching your baby and you will influence and soothe one another. If your baby is stressed, breathe deeply, find a relaxing spot, and relax ... if you are stressed, lie next to her while she is peaceful and breathe in her scent ... even a few minutes can make a world of difference.

Bonding

Everyone talks about bonding, but what does it mean? One definition is: falling in love. You may feel it before birth, or the sensation may sweep over you the minute you lay eyes on one another. Love hormones (page 74) naturally incline women to fall in love; and babies have their own supply. Even without the same quantities of these, men can be stirred to their deepest core. But bonding is not always automatic. Some mums and dads feel numb. The feeling may come after a good sleep following birth; once you have held your baby closely, skin to skin; in a few days when breastfeeding is established; or after a few weeks. Some parents are afraid to fall in love and some babies seem distant.

If you feel no bond, do talk to someone and consider some practical help to relieve stress. Many things affect bonding, including what happened during birth, your feelings about responsibility, your own early life experiences, and current relationships. Remember how powerful your baby is: in your two-way relationship you can receive as well as give. It is difficult to bond if you do not spend undisturbed quality time together.

'It's like she's always been here – now I can see her, I feel so much better. People say the first three months are the hardest but I've done the hardest part, I felt so ill in pregnancy. Now I feel better than I have done for a year. The thing is getting round to doing things like brushing my teeth ...'
Suzie

If the ride gets rocky

The ideal picture of love and bliss does not always happen; or it may alternate with uncertainty and tears. Many new parents feel shocked and exhausted, disorientated and confused. The prospect of caring for a dependent person may at times be overwhelming.

It is normal and OK to have less than happy feelings. Tiredness and the emotional tidal wave of birth can be draining, so expect ups and downs in the first days and weeks. This is usually most marked for mum, whose hormones fluctuate wildly.

Most people find that wonder overrides the negatives; but sometimes it can be the other way round. If you feel yourself going under:

▶ Talk to someone and arrange a break so you can rest.

▶ Spend time holding your baby, skin to skin, and looking into one another's eyes – this powerful communication switches on genes in both your brains that encourage bonding and relaxation. Try it in the bath.

▶ Dads often neglect their own needs. Make time for one-to-one with your baby and ask your partner to massage your hands, feet or head.

▶ If breastfeeding is difficult, you should seek support without delay.

▶ If breastfeeding is going well, use the time to relax, drink some water, and indulge in your baby.

▶ Let go of all but essential household chores: the dusting can wait.

▶ If either of you are feeling really blue, talk to a doctor or a healthcare professional you trust. Depression is common for men and for women after birth and passes more easily with support and loving guidance (see page 172). If your feelings continue, counselling might be very helpful.

Making eye contact with your baby is one of the simplest and most moving ways for you to tune into one another. From birth your baby can focus with complete clarity at a distance of around 30cm – the distance between a mother's breast and her face. He loves to look at your face.

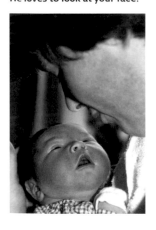

Now what do we do?

Unless you have experience with babies you may feel all fingers and thumbs … and you will be learning a new language as you decipher your baby's grimaces and cries. Relax and tune in – it doesn't take long before you find that caring for your baby will be second nature.

Contact

Your baby will want to smell, hear, feel and see you. Loving touch helps your baby to thrive. It helps her to grow, deepens the bond between you and relaxes you both. Using a papoose or sling is perfect when you're on the move. If your baby is in special care, you may be able to use kangaroo care (page 182); if not, touch through stroking is still beneficial.

Warmth

Newborn babies can't control their own body temperature: you need to do this. If you feel warm, so will your baby; if you are cold, she will be too. Remember, though, that body temperature rises when you are active and your baby does not move as much as you.

Dress her in soft, natural fabric clothes and use a cellular blanket when she sleeps. The number of layers depends on the air temperature. Your baby will be warmed by your body if you're holding her.

To check her temperature, feel her back and chest, not her hands or feet. If she is cold, she may cry and seem pale. She needs you to warm her by holding her; then add clothes or a blanket to help her maintain the heat if you're going to lie her separately. If she is too hot, she'll probably be flushed and may cry. Remove a layer of clothes; if it's a hot day, she may enjoy being naked.

> **watch out!**
>
> **Temperature warnings**
> You can take your baby's temperature with a non-invasive thermometer (e.g. one you place on her forehead). Call a doctor if her temperature is above 37 degrees, which indicates a fever, or below 35 degrees, which is dangerously low and she will require careful and gradual warming up.

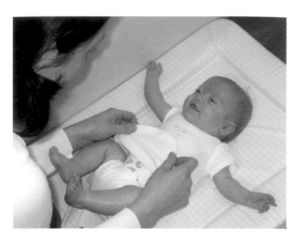

Nappies

Your midwife will guide you through your first nappy changes and you'll soon be doing them without thinking. Use changing times for playing and talking, making eye contact and soothing your baby. If she doesn't like it, be as quick as possible. If she's relaxed, let her lie with her skin exposed for a while.

▶ Change your baby's nappy roughly every three hours, sooner if it is swollen with urine, and immediately if she has passed a motion.

▶ At night, don't change her nappy if this will disturb her, unless it needs it.

▶ Which type of nappy? See page 36.

Nappy rash

Nappy rash is a blanket term for a variety of rashes that may be caused by something your baby has eaten (or what you eat if you're breastfeeding), by dirty nappies, by heat, teething, illness or infection, or by allergy. Angry red patches around the genitals, for instance, are probably a reaction to urine or faeces. White patches or spots surrounded by red starting at the anus and spreading over the buttocks may be caused by candida infection (page 170).

Guarding against nappy rash

▶ Keep your baby clean and dry. Use water and cotton wool to wash and natural oils to moisturize (page 39). Keep baby wipes for changes away from home and avoid heavily scented soaps.

▶ Give your baby time each day without a nappy on.

▶ Use a gentle detergent for washable nappies.

must know

Treatment for nappy rash
▶ Change nappies frequently, with time to air and dry your baby's skin.
▶ Use a soothing barrier cream like Sudocrem or Vaseline: apply it lightly, or it will trap moisture, and return to natural oils when the rash clears.
▶ Calendula creams and tinctures are soothing; acupressure can also help.
▶ Ask your midwife or health visitor to take a look.

▶ If your baby is given antibiotics she's more susceptible to candida; for some infections there may be gentler complementary treatment.

Baths

Your midwife may show you how to bath your baby. Many new parents find it a slippery and difficult business to begin with. You may enjoy sharing your bath; if you prefer to use a baby bath, cradle your baby safely; or you may kneel over your adult bath and rest your baby in a flannel support chair. Be gentle and reassuring as you lower your baby into the water. She may relax when she becomes weightless: some babies chill out so much, they sleep. If your baby howls, try sharing your bath; if that fails, stick to a gentle wipe down with cotton wool and water for the first few weeks. Have a warm towel ready.

Play

Your baby will enjoy stimulation, and will spend more time awake and respond with a greater range of movements as each week passes. Play is an important aspect of your relationship: it's also good for your baby's sense of delight and her development. The most entertaining thing for your baby is to watch your face. She'll also like physical play, beginning with very gentle massage and moving on to stretching and tickles. The authority on massaging is Peter Walker (www.thebabywebsite.com). You can use your own body as a gym.

Decorate your baby's pram, cot or play area. Go for bright, bold and contrasting patterns, and photos of faces. These help her brain and eyes develop, and seeing familiar faces will help her feel secure. Initially her head will rest to one side while she lies down: stick pictures where she will see them.

Don't leave your baby in her car seat when she's not in the car: the two best positions for strengthening her spine are to be held in a sling and to be laid flat on her back. It's also crucial to give her time on her tummy while she's awake. This develops her arm, shoulder and neck strength.

Feeding your baby

Breast milk is the best food for your baby. It comes at the perfect temperature, is full of antibodies, love hormones, vitamins, minerals and protein, and changes to meet her needs at each feed; and the contact is deeply pleasurable. Bottle feeding is a second best but still gives goodness and nutrition. Most parents begin with breast and, after weeks or months, move onto a bottle.

Breastfeeding

Your baby knows instinctively how to feed. You may find that she teaches you; sometimes the partnership works the other way and a mother needs to give guidance. Initially, you may appreciate some support from a midwife or breastfeeding specialist, since even with strong instincts and the best intentions seemingly small problems with positioning can lead to pain and difficulties. Taking care in the early days will help to set you both up for a blissful feeding partnership.

Breastfeeding basics

You and your baby will fare best if you are relaxed and undisturbed: try to create a calm atmosphere in the early days. When you've both settled in, you'll be more confident about feeding in different locations.

▶ Your baby's latching-on position is the most important factor. Your baby needs to suck on the red area around your nipple (your areola) and not on your nipple. Your baby's bottom lip needs to slip under your nipple. Your nipple points towards the roof of her mouth, and her top lip provides suction from above.

▶ Sit with back support and your feet flat on the ground or crossed if you sit on the floor. You can rest your baby on a pillow or cradle her in your arm and rest this on a cushion. You can also feed while lying down.

▶ Drink plenty of water to keep yourself hydrated and eat well – for your own energy and for good milk quality.

▶ Make sure you get enough rest.

▶ Use a bracelet to mark the side you start with; at the next feed, start from the other breast.

▶ Your baby will bring up milk in a 'posset' or with vomit. This doesn't affect her nutrition. If she does a projectile vomit on a number of occasions, let your doctor know. It's probably not a problem, but unusually can be caused by a condition that needs to be remedied surgically.

good to know

Is my baby getting enough?
Usually, the answer is yes. You can ask your health visitor to check weight gain. If you are worried because your baby cries a lot, there may be many causes besides hunger (pages 161–2).

When to feed

▶ Start as soon as you feel up to it. After a c-section a midwife may help you begin feeding in the recovery room.

▶ For at least five days after birth, feed on demand. Initially your breasts produce colostrum, which is bursting with goodness.

▶ Your milk will come in between day two and four, at which time your breasts are swollen and tender. Feed whenever your baby asks and encourage her to drain at least one, if not two, breasts. If she nods off, give her a gentle nudge or tickle her chin to help her continue sucking. A full feed will keep her satisfied for longer, and release the pressure on your breasts.

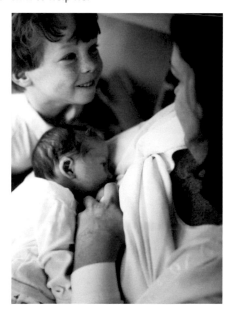

▶ Don't let your baby stay hungry or wail for her food: she needs to know you are there to meet her needs. If she's needy, she may gulp air and get painful wind.

▶ Your baby may feed at wide intervals; alternatively, she may be a grazer. Follow her rhythm. If you wish to introduce a routine of three- or four-hourly feeds, gradually move towards these intervals.

▶ You can express milk so your partner or someone else can feed your baby with a bottle: but don't do this until week eight or later as it could disrupt your flow.

watch out!

If your baby is not feeding
Ask a health carer to check your position and ask a doctor for advice. Difficulty feeding may occasionally be a sign that a baby is unwell and it is important to avoid dehydration and low blood sugar.

Common problems

Breastfeeding can be problem free. If something isn't right, though, take advice as soon as possible:

▶ Cracked nipples, perhaps bleeding: check your position and keep feeding. Don't let your baby chew on your nipple – her lips need to be around your areola with your nipple at the roof of her mouth. Nipple shields can help.

▶ Low milk flow: check your position, ensure you are eating and drinking well and are well rested. Feeling anxious, especially about your baby, may be a factor and things could improve if your concerns reduce.

▶ Engorgement (swollen, heavy breasts): feed your baby to release the pressure and check your position to ensure your baby is able to drain your breast. It may be painful but it's worth persisting. Gentle massage, from the rim of your breast to your nipple, working around your breast may help; as may expressing extra milk by hand or with a pump.

▶ Your baby complains: she may not like the taste. Think about what you've eaten recently. Strawberries and coffee are common culprits, but it could be anything.

▶ Your baby is very windy, or gags: alter her position or press your breast slightly at the start of a feed to reduce rapid flow. Let her rest and wind at intervals during a feed, if she wants to.

▶ Mastitis: this is an infection in the milk ducts, usually following engorgement. It needs antibiotic treatment.

See also www.breastfeedingnetwork.org.uk and www.laleche.org.uk.

When to stop breastfeeding

The current World Health Organization (WHO) recommendations state that exclusive breastfeeding for six months is optimal. Some people enjoy feeding for one, two or even three years, but for others, six months is difficult. While it's good to aim for a long period, if you don't manage six months, this is not a failure. You will have done your best. Even a few days of colostrum sets your baby up well.

The emotions of breastfeeding

Each time you breastfeed, you mix a hormonal cocktail that may make you ecstatic, dreamy, relaxed or even tearful. And the hormonal shift between feeds can do much the same thing. You may not feel quite like your 'old self' until you stop completely. And when you stop, you may get emotional again as your hormones change and you and your baby adjust to the separation.

'I expressed initially and Florence was fed in the special care unit. When we got together, I found it easy – she was a natural. The only time I needed guidance was at the six-week stage. My milk supply balanced for her needs, and I no longer felt really full. I worried I hadn't enough – in fact it was just the right amount. They don't tell you any of that in the hospital.'
Becca

Bottle feeding

Unless you breastfeed exclusively for the first year, you will need to bottle feed at some stage. The greatest bonus is that someone other than you can enjoy feeding and spending time with your baby as she relaxes into his feed.

Bottles from birth

If you have chosen to bottle feed from birth, think through your decision carefully: breast milk delivers goodness that your baby cannot get from formula. Even a few days at the breast is a bonus. Unusually, bottle feeding is essential because of health concerns.

Practicalities

▶ Follow the manufacturer's instructions carefully and always use boiled and cooled water.
▶ From birth, mix 50–75ml (2–3fl oz) at a feed and offer the bottle on demand. Your baby may take only 40ml (1½fl oz).
▶ By three months your baby may be taking 125–200ml (4–7fl oz) and going for up to four hours between feeds.

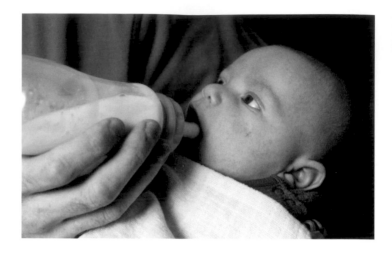

▶ Heat the bottle gently in a pan of water over the stove. Don't use a microwave.

▶ Shake the bottle well and test the milk temperature on the inside of your wrist – a little warmer than body temperature is perfect.

▶ Hold your baby so her head is slightly higher than her tummy, and angle the bottle so she doesn't guzzle or gulp air.

▶ Find a system that suits you so that you always have sterilized bottles to hand. You can mix a few bottles in advance and keep them in the fridge.

Mixing breast and bottle

If you want to combine breast and bottle, hold back until you have been feeding for eight weeks, by which time your breasts will be used to their new role. Some people choose to use one bottle at night – maybe a feed for dad to enjoy.

Your baby may take to the bottle with ease, or may refuse it. She might also be happier to take it from someone other than you (you smell of sumptuous milk).

must know

What you will need
▶ At least eight bottles with newborn teats and lids.
▶ A sterilizing kit – you can boil or steam your bottles on the stove but electrical kits are less hassle.
▶ Newborn formula milk – organic is available.
▶ A few babies react to one or other formula with symptoms such as wind, constipation, rashes or bottle rejection. Consult your doctor if you're concerned. If you wish to use non-dairy milk, take advice to ensure your baby is getting the goodness she needs.

Crying: what is your baby telling you?

Babies have an incredible range of cries with different rhythms and pitches to convey specific messages. The language is so primal, and so emotional, that it resonates with your body and often gets just the response that's needed. Not all crying is a call for help, though. Your baby openly expresses the way she feels and sometimes she may need to 'let it all out' ... she will be able to do this best if you are there for her.

Tuning in

You will soon get to know your baby's language, although your understanding is unlikely to come overnight and sometimes you won't be able to soothe her quickly. Don't panic. It can take time to tune in, and you may be relieved to know that it's quite normal for newborn babies to cry for a total of six hours in a 24-hour period.

If you're at a loss for how to soothe your baby, remember that crying is only one aspect of her language: you may be able to gain more clues about the way she is feeling from her facial expressions and other body movements. Finally, look after yourself. It really is OK to hand over to someone else and to take a break.

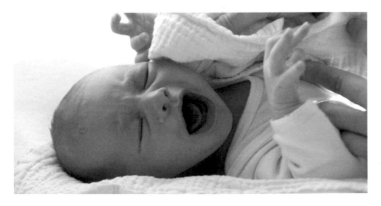

Why your baby might cry

Why might your baby cry?	What can you try?
She needs you	Hold her, put down what you are doing and be there for her
Hungry	Try feeding; if she's really wailing, rock and calm her before beginning the feed
Wind or tummy pain	She may suckle initially, then cry again; hold her on your shoulder or rest her over your lap to wind her
Other pain, e.g. head	She may feel pain if there was pressure as she was born and almost certainly if forceps or ventouse were used; try massage, osteopathy, holding
Anger or shock, perhaps as a reaction to birth	Talk to her, tell her you are listening, rock her in your arms, play music you played in pregnancy, try massage or osteopathy
Too hot or too cold	Warm or cool her (see page 153)
Time to poo	She may be more comfortable if you hold her upright on your shoulder
Tired	Dim the lights, help her relax, take your baby for a walk in a sling or pram, or lie her down to sleep, ensuring she is swaddled and warm
Bored	Talk to and play with your baby
'Crying time' – this is often early evening	Take time to soothe and calm her, maybe walking around with her; a ride in the car may help but don't make this a daily habit – it'll be hard to break
Picking up on anxiety in home	It may help to address anxiety or conflict in yourself or at home; for tips, turn to page 18
Illness	Ask a healthcare professional for advice

watch out!

Red alert

If your baby's cry is high-pitched and unusual, this may be a sign of pain. If your stomach lurches, your instinct's telling you something isn't right. Take her to a doctor.

Leaving her to cry

You cannot spoil your baby – she simply expresses her feelings and asks for comfort. Don't leave her to cry as a matter of course: if her cries are regularly unanswered she may learn that her needs won't be easily met and this may affect her behaviour in relationships and her self-esteem for years to come. Once in a while, though, being left for a few minutes may be best for all of you if you need a break.

Sleep

Babies need to sleep a lot: it's an essential part of their development. While your baby sleeps she integrates her feelings and the enormous amount she is learning as she rests and dreams. Initially, you need to adapt to her rhythm because she will sleep when she needs to; in time, she will adapt to yours and you can introduce a routine.

Comfort

A full tummy, no wind, a clean nappy, warmth and company usually add up to a happy baby, ready to slumber. If your baby seems tired but cannot sleep, check that all these essentials are in place. Some babies prefer to be quiet and undisturbed; some prefer to be rocked and carried.

Family sleeping

Comfort involves being close to you. No other mammal sleeps apart from their newborn babies, and it's best for your baby if she sleeps in your room for at least three months. She'll be reassured and you'll all be less disturbed when you wake to feed. You could have a Moses basket or cot next to your bed.

The WHO advises against sleeping with your baby in your bed as a safety precaution but there are well-researched views countering this advice. Many parents relish the delightful intimacy of sharing a bed and say that it reduces rather than increases sleep disruption, and makes for a happier baby and easier parenting. (For more information, see *Three in a Bed* by Deborah Jackson.)

> **watch out!**
>
> **Sudden infant death syndrome (SIDS)**
> SIDS is a worry for most parents, even though 1:1600 babies is affected. Precautionary measures include:
> ► Lie your baby on her back in the 'feet to foot' position in her cot, so her feet reach the bottom. Her head may be several inches from the top. This is to prevent her wriggling down beneath the bedclothes.
> ► Make sure your baby is neither too hot nor too cold (see page 153).
> ► Sleep with your baby in your room. When you are not with her, use a monitor.
> ► Never smoke around your baby.
> ► Never sleep with your baby if you have taken drugs, sedatives or alcohol.

The red-eye life

Feeling tired is usual but there are ways to reduce or avoid exhaustion. Sleeping with or near your baby is one way. If you find it difficult to sleep, try a breathing exercise or visualization. During the day, catch up on sleep when you can. Resting in yoga poses can be extremely revitalizing (see page 83). It's also worth sharing the load so one of you can get a good sleep in a spare room or on the sofa: if you're breastfeeding, your partner or another helper can bring baby to you and then settle her after her feed.

Sleepy time

Initially, your baby will sleep for 16–20 out of every 24 hours, at intervals of 30 minutes to three hours. She will gradually spend more time awake. Between the hours of 8pm and 8am your new baby may wake three to six times.

Regular patterns of feeding and sleeping help your baby to thrive but strict timetables do not suit a new baby. The key is to work around your baby's rhythms and gently guide her: she will at times need help to relax and fall asleep. With respect for her needs you can, over a number of weeks, help her sleep at times that suit her as well as you. You may find that your rhythms are in harmony from the beginning.

When she's sleeping lightly, your baby may grumble for a minute or two then go back to sleep of her own accord. If she wails, she needs you and it's important to go to her even if her pattern has changed from yesterday or last week – every baby will become upset if left to cry in a room on her own when she really needs her parents. Bear this in mind if you wish to help your baby settle into a routine.

Some babies love to be swaddled while they sleep: it gives a feeling of security and stops a baby from waking herself up as she fidgets.

Into the future

As each day passes, your baby grows and brings something new to your life. Look after yourself, your baby and your relationship, and you'll be doing the best possible for you all.

One day at a time

You can make the most of the precious early days by spending lots of time with your baby, resting when you can, eating well and being with other adults and new parents. Exercise gently and take time to chill: even ten minutes' peace can make a huge difference.

Take it one day at a time: small adjustments depending on what's happening for each one of you will help you to keep a balance and nurture your baby and yourselves in this exciting new stage of your lives.

'If there's one thing I would tell people who are having a baby, it is this. After birth at the end of three months you finally have time to talk to one another again. It's like you need to work out who you are as individuals, and where your relationship is after the arrival of a new person. After my third baby, I realized this, but after the first two we were both thrown off course. Being prepared makes it so much easier to move forward in a good way.'
Gabi

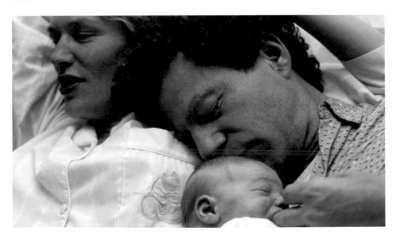

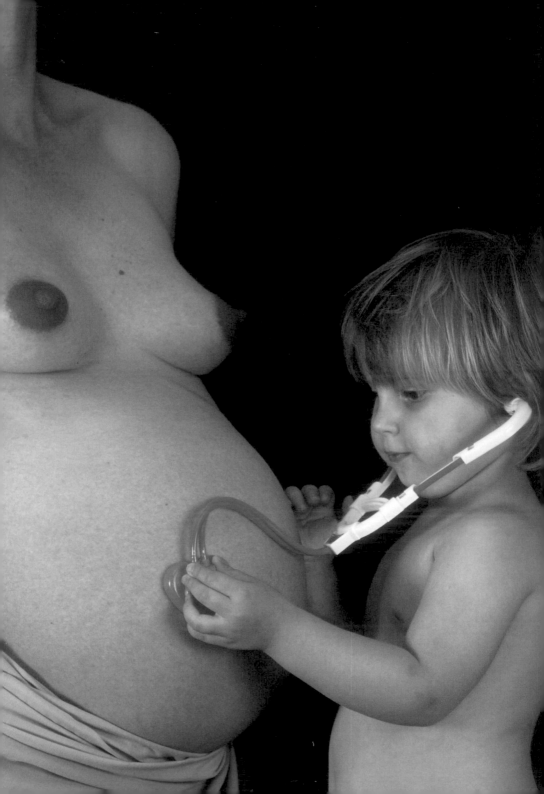

6 A–Z of health concerns

Beyond minor niggles and unpleasant symptoms that pass with time, most pregnancies go without serious problems. Yet pregnancy is a time of questions and, sometimes, anxiety that all might not be well. This section gives an overview of the pregnancy-specific issues most commonly faced by expectant parents. Usually, diagnosis and medical or complementary treatment measures are straightforward. Rarely, a serious issue is detected; if this happens, you may choose to have specialist support. The A-Z entries in the following pages are intended as your first point of reference. For further details, please use the books and websites listed on pages 187–9.

Abdominal pain

If your pain is severe, see your doctor; certainly if you have any bleeding. If your pain is moderate, don't worry. It's probably due to muscle tension and softened ligaments, or may be caused by wind. Talk to your midwife at your next visit and follow the ABC (page 19). In late pregnancy, Braxton-Hicks contractions may be painful. **Unlikely causes:** *ectopic pregnancy, miscarriage, placental abruption.* **See also** *Pain in pregnancy.*

Amniotic fluid: too much (polyhydramnios)

This probably reflects your pregnancy and your baby's size, with no cause for concern. You may feel a little breathless and your baby may find it more comfortable to lie bottom down (breech) or across your abdomen (tranverse). Your team will want to monitor the level as severe polyhydramnios may trigger *premature labour and birth*: resting may reduce this risk. **Rarely** a baby has difficulty swallowing and passing the fluid.

Amniotic fluid: too little (oligohydramnios)

This is probably no cause for concern. Your baby's growth will be monitored in case there is a link with *intra-uterine growth restriction (IUGR)* and poor placental function, although this is unusual. In labour, low levels may increase the risk of foetal distress. Early

induction or a caesarean may be considered.

Anaemia

Don't worry. You have low levels of iron in your blood, which might make you tired and low and perhaps faint, but there's no risk to your baby. You're more susceptible if you are carrying twins or a large baby and if you usually have heavy periods or IBS. The most common cause is vitamin and mineral deficiency, usually iron. Follow the ABC (page 19). Almonds, apricots, coriander, seaweed and spinach are all rich in iron and you could take an extra supplement: iron with vitamin C one hour before eating. The rare inherited conditions sickle cell disease and thalassaemia require specialist care.

Anxiety and stress

Rare indeed are women and men who don't feel some anxiety and/or stress in pregnancy. Anxiety might trigger or exacerbate other symptoms, such as nausea, *diarrhoea, constipation*, pain, insomnia, cravings, vivid dreams and also further anxiety. If prolonged, anxiety increases the likelihood of complications in labour, and may cause your baby to be irritable after birth. So it's important to do what you can to relax your mind and body. **See also** page 18.

Back pain

In pregnancy, this is probably due to normal changes in your spine and pelvis, ligaments and muscles. It's not a sign of a serious problem, nor does it make discomfort in labour more likely. It may, however, put a downer on things. Take heart; there are many ways to alleviate it, including attention to your posture (page 100), stress relief and physiotherapy and other complementary therapies (page 000). If pain does not reduce, get extra practical help so you can rest. **After birth,** the pains of pregnancy tend to pass: back pain is usually the result of the new demands of holding, rocking and feeding a baby. If you have had an epidural, back pain is a possible side effect. For more, look at the tips for relieving pain (page 112). **See also** www.pregnancy.com.au/back_pain.

Bleeding in pregnancy

Vaginal bleeding is not necessarily a sign of trouble but you must be checked as soon as possible. Experiencing bleeding is quite possibly one of the most frightening symptoms: if you're on your own, call someone to be with you. Remember, it is always important to be checked medically, even if bleeding is light. If bleeding is heavy and you are in pain, this is an emergency. **First trimester (weeks 1–12):** light 'implantation' bleeding (spotting) is relatively common in the first six weeks and carries no risk to your baby. Heavy bleeding may pass and is a 'threatened miscarriage' if your cervix is not dilating. You'll be advised to rest and abstain from sex; it may be necessary to stay in hospital. In seven out of ten instances, pregnancy continues to full term. If you bleed heavily with clots and pain, and your cervix is dilating, this may be *miscarriage*. **Second and third trimesters (weeks 13–40):** light, bright red bleeding could arise from a *vaginal infection*; or the blood may be coming from your cervix ('cervical erosion') and there is no risk to your baby; or it may signal *placenta praevia*, which could necessitate caesarean delivery. Close to term a small amount of blood may be a 'show' before the onset of labour (page 117); it's often mixed with mucus. Dark blood, probably with pain, is potentially serious and could arise because of *placental abruption*: in most cases an emergency caesarean is essential. Heavy blood with clots may be a sign of late miscarriage. After week 20, loss is a *still birth*. After week 26, bleeding could mark the onset of *premature labour*.

Blood pressure: high (hypertension) and pre-eclampsia

In pregnancy, high blood pressure (BP) is called pre-eclampsia. Mildly raised blood pressure is seldom a concern but very high pressure carries a risk of bleeding and *placental abruption* and, in labour, increases the risk of foetal distress. If you have high BP as well as protein in your urine, your midwife will want to monitor you closely. Follow the ABC (page 19), remembering that stress, overdoing things could raise your blood pressure. Try breathing exercises at least twice a day. You may be advised to give birth in a hospital with facilities for c-section and epidural (which can lower blood pressure). Occasionally, medication is used, and sometimes it is safer to induce labour before full term. **Rare conditions:** eclampsia, where prolonged high BP affects the brain, causing convulsions. Early treatment of high BP almost always prevents this.

Blood pressure: low (hypotension)

Low blood pressure is a sign of good health. The down side is that you may feel light headed or faint. If you do, move around to get your circulation going. As you stand, hold on to something and tighten and release the muscles in your calves, thighs and buttocks two or three times. Low blood pressure is not a risk for your baby except in the rare circumstance that it follows heavy blood loss: in this case you may need a blood transfusion.

Breast pain

Your breasts change throughout pregnancy and might be uncomfortable. Wearing a supportive bra will help: move up a size as you need, and try a sports bra at night. Gentle massage, from the edge to the nipple, may ease your pain. **After birth,** discomfort is linked to milk flow: attention to your baby's position offers the best resolution (page 156). If there is

an infection – mastitis – antibiotics are recommended.

Candida (thrush)

Candida is common in pregnancy when vaginal sugar and acidity levels provide a friendly environment for the bacteria. If you have had frequent infections in the past, you're more vulnerable. Ask a doctor to confirm the infection. For comfort advice, see page 73. Recurrent thrush may be a manifestation of emotional or sexual issues arising from previous trauma: counselling may bring relief.

Carpal tunnel syndrome

Extra fluid in your circulation may compress the median nerve in your wrist, causing pain in your fingers. Gently massage your wrists, concentrating on the joint closest to the back of your hand. Sleep with your hands raised on your pillow and in the day try gently stretching by resting on all fours for a minute or two with your hands flat, fingers facing your knees. Your doctor may give you a wrist splint.

Cervical incompetence

Your cervix is kept closed by muscles that soften before labour. Around 1:100 women have an incompetent cervix. Unfortunately, the first sign is usually a second trimester *miscarriage* because the muscles are not strong enough to hold the cervix closed. In a future pregnancy, a stitch can be inserted in weeks 12–16, and removed around week 36. Labour usually follows within two to four weeks.

Chicken pox

If you are not immune and you come into contact with chicken pox, tell your midwife. If you become infected, you might pass the infection to your baby and there is a small risk that this could affect growth. The risk is greatest before week 20. If you're infected within days of birth, your baby will be checked by a paediatrician for neonatal chicken pox. Shingles has no effect for a baby.

Chlamydia

Chlamydia is the most common sexually transmitted disease but 85% of infected people do not know they carry the bacteria because symptoms are rare (e.g. fever, bleeding, pain on urination and yellowish *vaginal discharge*; men can experience discharge and pain). **Infection in pregnancy** could trigger premature birth and conjunctivitis for a baby; for a woman it can reduce future fertility. You and your partner need to be treated with antibiotics. Eat live yoghurt or take probiotic tablets, which reduce susceptibility to side effects like *diarrhoea* and *candida* (*thrush*).

Cholestasis

Cholestasis only occurs in pregnancy and affects around 1:100 women. Severe itching, mostly on the palms of your hands and soles of your feet, arises when your liver's bile production is abnormal. It's most common after week 30. Calomine lotion may relieve itching. Cholestasis increases your baby's susceptibility to foetal distress in labour, and doubles the likelihood of *premature labour and birth*. Medical treatment usually involves taking bile acid in tablet form; it should reduce itching within 48 hours but may cause mild *diarrhoea*. You may be given *vitamin K* weekly to improve your blood's clotting ability. If your bile salt levels remain high, your birth team may recommend induction around weeks 37–38.

Congenital abnormalities

Any aspect of development that varies from the norm is a congenital ('born with') abnormality. In most cases there is little impact but occasionally the under-lying abnormality – whether genetic or developmental – may affect health for years. **Rarely**, it is life threatening. Around two-thirds of abnormalities are detected in pregnancy; the remainder become apparent either at birth or in the weeks or months that follow. If an abnormality is suspected in pregnancy because you have a family history or a scan suggests a problem, a diagnostic test such as amniocentesis is recommended. If you learn that your baby is affected in some way, you may face challenging decisions. An obstetrician or genetic counsellor will support you. You may also want to talk to an independent counsellor. Some conditions can be relieved or resolved in pregnancy and/or after birth. Sometimes, operating is the best option, e.g. heart or stomach problems. You will be guided by a specialist paediatrician and nurses. **Forward planning**: one of the most positive things you can do is to plan support now and after the birth or following a termination, if this is your choice. Emotionally you are likely to be shocked and confused, with mood swings, pain and sadness. There may be extra care available in your community. Sometimes getting the care you are entitled to takes energy and persistence: you may need someone to help you fill in forms and cut through the red tape. Local and national groups can be a life line. **See also** antenatal screening and testing (pages 49–53); *Down's syndrome*; *special care*; *premature labour and birth*; www.scope.org.uk.

Constipation

Constipation is defined as the absence of stools for three or more days or the passing of unusually hard stools, but there is a wide variation as to what brings discomfort. A number of things may bring on constipation: these include pregnancy hormones, what you eat, IBS, your lifestyle and how you feel emotionally (especially if you're nervous, stressed or holding back from expressing something). Follow the ABC (page 19), focusing on your diet. You need adequate fibre and plenty

of water. You may need to change your iron supplement. Linseeds are the most effective natural laxatives and homeopathy might help. You may notice changes within a week or two. Your midwife may recommend a bulk laxative.

Depression

In pregnancy, depression is common and after birth as many as eight in ten women feel mildly depressed. Fewer feel severely depressed. Men are also susceptible to pre- and postnatal depression.

There is no single reason. Hormonal changes play a role for women but are seldom the sole cause. After birth, the demands of parenting and disturbed sleep are both significant, and how you felt during labour and birth are very influential. Parenthood may also make you anxious and changes to your relationship, lifestyle and work may be upsetting. Depression can involve grief – and many parents feel they have lost a part of themselves despite the gain of a new baby. What has happened in your past also contributes to how you feel now. The transition into parenthood brings up buried emotions and many feelings may be confusing.

Take heart that if you feel down you have not failed, nor done anything wrong. It is OK to admit your feelings and talking about them as well as asking for practical help or emotional guidance is a good way to strengthen yourself as you set out on the road to parenthood. This is a new life stage and it may take time for you to find your feet as you adjust to the physical and emotional changes. Occasionally medication is helpful but you need to consider the pros and cons. Follow the advice on page 20 and consider seeing a homeopath, whose remedies will support you emotionally at the same time as addressing your pregnancy symptoms/postnatal recovery. You may also wish to see a counsellor or psychotherapist – therapists specializing in early parenting issues will be happy to see you with your baby. If you feel you are completely losing control or have urges to harm or neglect yourself or your baby, do talk to your doctor. The **rare condition** puerperal psychosis requires specialist medical care.

Diabetes

If you are diabetic and your blood sugar levels are carefully controlled you may not experience any unusual symptoms or difficulties. The risks of complications, though, are higher: these reflect the extent of your blood sugar fluctuation. Your specialist and midwife will monitor you closely. Occasionally, diabetes occurs for the first time in pregnancy, as 'gestational diabetes'. There may be no symptoms apart from blood in your urine, or you may feel tired, dizzy, hungry or confused. The key to keeping your blood sugar stable is your diet. Eat well and regularly, but ensure you don't have too many calories as you are vulnerable to gaining extra weight. Exercise also helps. Use the ABC (page 19). If you have Type I diabetes, you will need to continue taking extra insulin. **See also** www.diabetes.org.uk; there may be a pregnancy diabetic clinic at your hospital.

Diarrhoea

Although diarrhoea can be triggered by an intolerance to food or by *anxiety*, it usually arises from infection. Your midwife may recommend a stool test, with treatment advice depending on the results. Drink plenty of water to guard against dehydration. To replace lost electrolytes and other nutrients, drink rehydration formulae, which are available from chemists. When you feel like eating again, begin with bananas, white rice or white toast. Bio-yoghurt will help to repopulate your intestine with 'friendly' bacteria. Gradually introduce foods without fat. If you don't have an infection, you may be sensitive to a specific food, or to a combination of foods, and underlying IBS may be a factor. Your habits may have changed – are you drinking more fruit juice or eating less fibre, for instance? **In pre-labour** diarrhoea is common when hormones stimulate your bowel to contract.

Down's syndrome

Down's syndrome is an uncommon condition that affects physical and mental development. It is the most frequently detected *congenital abnormality* in pregnancy, usually caused by a triple – rather than a double – set of the 21st chromosome in each cell. Mothers below 25 years have an average risk of a Down's syndrome pregnancy of about 1:1400. The risk rises to about 1:350 at 35 and 1:40 at age 43 years. People with Down's syndrome have a reputation for being loving and enthusiastic; but the condition may impede hearing, vision, speech and movement, and increases susceptibility to illness. It also affects mental acuity, and a child with Down's syndrome may find it difficult to learn to express what she is feeling and to read emotions in others. **See also** antenatal testing (page 000); *congenital abnormalities*; www.altonweb.com/cs/downsyndrome/index.htm.

Ectopic pregnancy

The first sign of an ectopic pregnancy is usually sharp *pain* on one side of the abdomen; this may be accompanied by *bleeding*. This is an emergency. In an ectopic pregnancy, the egg settles outside your uterus, probably in a fallopian tube. It happens in 1:100 pregnancies (more with IVF). Except in extremely rare circumstances, an ectopic pregnancy cannot continue. Your doctor will assess what's happening with the assistance of ultrasound scanning. Your body may reabsorb the pregnancy over

four to ten weeks, but if there is internal bleeding, an operation is essential, either a laparoscopy (via your umbilicus) or a laparotomy (an incision in your abdomen). Pain and loss bring intense emotions and you may need a lot of support. Sometimes the emotional impact does not become apparent for weeks or months. Following an ectopic pregnancy, around 80% of women celebrate normal pregnancy: the chances are highest if you do not need surgery. **See also** www.womens-health.co.uk/ectopic.asp.

Fibroids

Fibroids do not occur for the first time in pregnancy, but existing fibroids may enlarge and can cause pain. A fibroid is a thickening of the uterine muscle tissue on or in the uterine wall or inside the uterine cavity. Follow the ABC (page 19) and try homeopathy to make symptoms less troublesome. Your fibroids may not interfere with a vaginal birth. If they are large, however, and your baby has chosen an awkward position, a caesarean section may be safest. **After birth,** there is a risk your fibroids may bleed and hinder the birth of the placenta. Your midwife may recommend an oxytocin injection to speed up delivery (page 131).

Fits and epilepsy

It is reassuring that over 90% of women with epilepsy have completely normal pregnancies. But an epileptic fit during pregnancy may cause *placental abruption* or premature rupture of the membranes (page 102). Your midwife and specialist carers will be able to advise you on preventative measures. Medication can harm a baby so you need specialist advice to minimize the risks particularly in the first ten weeks. If you have a fit in late pregnancy, you may need an emergency caesarean.

Headaches

Headaches are common and usually reflect physical pregnancy changes, emotional, sleep and lifestyle issues, or a cold. Because there is a small chance a headache could indicate an underlying problem such as pre-eclampsia, tell your midwife, and call your doctor if you have a sudden or severe headache. Posture is often the root cause. Your diet is important too – headache can accompany low blood sugar. Follow the ABC (page 19). You can take Paracetamol (one to two every four hours, up to four tablets in 24 hours) but addressing the underlying cause is best. Osteopathy often brings relief. After birth, if you have an epidural, a headache may persist for a few days or weeks.

Herpes

Don't worry if you have been infected in the past and do not have vaginal sores now: this presents no risks. Nor is herpes infection on the mouth an issue. There is only a potential (and small) risk if you have an active genital infection when you give birth; or if you become infected for the first time in pregnancy. Around 1:44,000 babies is affected and requires treatment after birth. If you are infected, stay clean and comfortable. The sores will pass. Try homeopathy and use tea tree oil in a bath to soothe the area. Anti-viral medication has not been cleared for use in pregnancy. Syphillis is rare but on the rise, with symptoms that mimic herpes.

HIV

HIV (human immunodeficiency virus) affects and undermines the immune system. It is responsible for acquired immune deficiency syndrome (AIDS) but does not always manifest as AIDS: current treatments mean HIV is more often a chronic illness than a fatal condition. HAART - 'highly active antiretroviral therapy' - greatly reduces susceptibility to infections. If you are infected, you can have a baby and be healthy enough to raise your baby and look forward to many years together. In pregnancy, the risk of passing the infection to your baby is relatively low: 2% born to HIV+ mothers are infected when medication is used. If you feel normal and healthy, the greatest effect is likely to be the emotional impact of the illness for you and for your family; and perhaps side effects from medication. You will need to take specialist advice about preventing transmission (e.g.

delivery by caesarean; avoiding breastfeeding). **After birth** it may be several months before tests can confirm that your baby is not affected; this is a difficult time. You will all benefit from support. **Must know:** HIV is not transmitted from a father to a developing baby. If you have no evidence of HIV infection now and when you are tested again in three months, your baby will not be infected.

Incontinence

In pregnancy, mild urinary leakage is common, particularly when you cough, sneeze, laugh or run. Your hormones relax the muscles and ligaments in your bladder, vagina and pelvic floor. Anal incontinence affects fewer women. Both are more likely after birth, usually temporarily. The key is to exercise your pelvic floor muscles regularly (page 81). Sex is also excellent exercise. Use a thin panty liner to stay fresh and follow the ABC (page 19), remembering that eating well supports healthy tissues. **After birth** if your nerves are bruised or your muscles have stretched a great deal, it may be difficult to tighten the area. Physiotherapy and vaginal cones may help and electrical stimulation may be recommended to gradually tone your muscles. **Rarely** the vaginal walls lose their tone and drop down after birth, in vaginal prolapse. The effect may not be apparent for several months but the vagina usually returns to normal.

Indigestion and heartburn

In pregnancy, the acidic, burning feeling of indigestion is common. It does not signify a problem and tends to settle after birth. It's partly due to the relaxation of muscles and valves in your oesophagus (food tube) and stomach. **To help,** be observant about food that affects you most. Citrus fruits do it for some people; wheat, coffee or dairy products do it for others. Some women swear by antacid medication for temporary relief. Keep your meal portions moderate and avoid smoking, fizzy drinks, caffeine and alcohol. Try not to slouch, and at night sleep propped up. A gentle abdominal massage with lemon or ginger oil may help. Mint tea is a traditional soother.

Intra-uterine growth restriction (IUGR)

This is the term used if your baby is growing at a rate attained by fewer than 5% of babies at the same stage of pregnancy. Your baby's size is estimated by your midwife and measured more accurately using ultrasound. Apparent slow growth may not indicate any significant problems. Most babies who are 'small for dates' are genetically programmed to be small and are growing perfectly normally. Your baby's growth may indicate how supportive his environment is, and there may be ways to improve this. Growth also provides information about vulnerability during labour. There may be no apparent cause, even though some influences (such as smoking or high blood pressure) are known. On a small number of occasions a baby with IUGR may have a genetic or developmental problem (page 172). You will be monitored closely through pregnancy. **During labour,** your baby may have fewer energy stores and become distressed more easily. If IUGR is severe, a caesarean might be advised before full term, or if it's moderate, your team may suggest induction towards full term. **After birth,** most IUGR babies show no problems but because being small is a slight disadvantage feed as soon as you feel ready, and then feed on demand. Keep your baby warm and hold her skin to skin or massage her frequently, as touch stimulates growth hormones. IUGR babies are more likely to develop jaundice. If your baby needs treatment, he will lie under a special light next to your bed. If your baby is born prematurely or has a *congenital abnormality*, he may need additional assistance in a *special care* unit.

Itching and rashes

Itching is very common, usually on the abdomen and most intensely in the last ten weeks. It tends to disappear after birth. Rashes are also common and are often unexplained. Usually there is no cause for concern. The main problem is if itching becomes excruciating and/or stops you from sleeping. Follow the ABC

(page 19) and for comfort try aloe vera lotion, calomine or other natural oils or creams. Wear light, natural fibres and use cotton bedclothes. Homeopathic remedies may be the best treatment. If itching is so bad that you are at the end of your tether and close to term, your birth team may recommend medication or induction. Because a rash may signal an infection it is important to have a medical examination. Itching may be linked with *cholestasis*.

Large babies

Around 10:100 babies are at least 4kg (8lb 12oz) at birth: this is large or 'macrosomic'. Being large may not present any problems although it may make birth difficult for your baby and increase your risk of tearing. A lot depends on your body build, the size of your pelvis, and how labour progresses. Many people celebrate the arrival of a large baby without any complications. The main concern is slow progress in the first stage of labour (page 130). In the second stage it will help if you are upright. **Rarely** larger size increases the risk that a baby's shoulder becomes stuck after his head is born ('shoulder dystocia'). This requires expert obstetric care to ensure safe delivery.

Miscarriage

If you are bleeding heavily and your cervix is dilating, this is a true miscarriage. It is usually very painful.

You may wish to stay at home and let the loss continue naturally. There will be pain and bleeding for 8–36 hours. You may prefer to stay in hospital for an operation (D&C) that clears your uterus. Women who miscarry at home sometimes need a D&C to protect against pain and infection. Miscarriage is a devastating loss; usually felt more acutely by women than by their partners. Almost all feel hurt, shocked and sad. Guilt is also common, particularly if pregnancy was not wanted. Having the company and love of your partner and/or a close friend may help you process your feelings. Grieving may continue for weeks or months, or begin years later. **After a miscarriage,** your body, mind and spirit integrate the loss. You need to avoid strenuous exercise for four to six weeks. Having people around who can help you rest and eat well will be an enormous help and you may want to use complementary therapies. Sometimes the best healing comes from sharing experiences. Talk to your midwife or try the internet for information on local and national miscarriage support groups.

Nausea and vomiting

Nausea is very common in the first stage of pregnancy – 70% of women feel sick, and many vomit occasionally or every day. It usually passes by week 12–16. Morning sickness presents no risk to your baby. Your sickness may be worse when you eat certain foods, at specific times of day, when you feel anxious or if you become tired. **To help,** follow the ABC (page 19). Muscle tension may also contribute: consider a massage. After vomiting, rinse your mouth out with water or use a natural mouth wash. Stomach acids weaken tooth enamel and frequent brushing could cause erosion. **Rarely** severe vomiting occurs: Hyperemesis requires rest and treatment in hospital.

Osteoporosis

Pregnancy is not a cause of osteoporosis. In pregnancy, your bones tend to absorb more calcium, which is a good thing, although they may lose density while breastfeeding. Preventative measures are important: consume a balance of calcium and other minerals with vitamin D (needed for calcium absorption); avoid carbonated drinks and high quantities of sugar; reduce red meat and hard cheese (whose acidity can cause your bones to leach calcium); and exercise regularly – walking, yoga and pilates are all great for your bones. There's more on eating well on page 20.

Pain in pregnancy

Pregnancy often entails aches and pains. Though these rarely signal a serious problem, you must seek urgent medical attention if: there is an intense or sudden onset of severe pain in your abdomen or pelvis; you have abdominal pain accompanied by vaginal *bleeding*; or abdominal pain with shivering; intense pain in your head with dizziness and/or disturbed vision; intense pain and swelling in your leg; or severe chest pain and breathlessness.

If you are in pain, tell your midwife or consultant, even if you think your pain is trivial. If an underlying condition is identified (e.g. infection), treatment is likely to bring relief; occasionally a condition cannot be easily treated but professional care helps to minimize discomfort. Many women find that complementary therapies offer the most powerful relief.

For relief you can take Paracetamol (one to two every four hours, up to four tablets in 24 hours) as a short-term option. But addressing the underlying cause is most effective. It's important to talk to your doctor about your requirements and the safety issues. Your posture can make a big difference (page 100). Depending on your pain, gentle walking or swimming may help, as may yoga, but you do need to take sufficient rest too, as being tired increases your pain sensitivity and muscle tension.

Your emotions may contribute to your tension and discomfort: working through fears or difficult feelings could help more than you expect – perhaps also with a knock-on effect on your posture, energy levels and motivation to exercise. Sensitivity to one or more foods, going hungry, eating too much or a high-sugar diet can all trigger or exacerbate pain. You may be surprised that eating regular nutritious meals helps.

Breathing deep and regularly relieves tension and pain; you could combine it with visualization (page 91). Complementary therapies that may help include acupuncture, homeopathy, massage and osteopathy (see page 47) You may be referred to a physiotherapist if you have back or *pelvic pain*.

Pelvic pain (SPD)

Pain in the pelvis that makes it uncomfortable to open your legs, get in or out of the car, or even walk, may be due to symphysis pubis dysfunction (SPD). Usually, this arises because of exaggerated opening of a joint called the pubic symphysis. Follow the advice for pain and be careful to avoid opening your legs wide. Roll over onto your side and get up very carefully from bed or the bath, or when you lie on the floor; seek advice if you are practising yoga or pilates; and avoid breaststroke if you swim. Cranial osteopathy is one of the most powerful treatments, although pain may not pass completely until after birth when the gap decreases. Your supporting ligaments take three to five months to get back to normal, so continue to be cautious about the way you move.

Piles (haemorrhoids)

Piles are not dangerous, simply unpleasant. They are very common, caused by swollen veins in the anus. Piles may be smaller than a pea, but can grow to the size of a grape. You may notice mucus discharge or bright red blood when you poo; and your anal muscle may go into spasm. Your doctor can detect piles with a finger-examination: to see very small piles she may use a small instrument. Don't stand for too long if this is uncomfortable, and use a cushion or a rubber ring to sit comfortably. Avoid foods that cause constipation, and drink at least 2 litres (3½ pints) of water a day. Pelvic floor exercises (page 81) will support circulation and reduce swelling. suppositories may help. Cortisone cream contains a mild anaesthetic and can reduce muscle spasm: your doctor can prescribe this. **After birth,** piles tend to settle down or disappear completely within 6–12 weeks. **Rarely** piles do not improve after birth and an operation may be recommended to remove them.

Placenta accreta

Placental accreta is a very rare occurrence where the placenta grows through the muscle wall of the uterus. This is not a problem in pregnancy but after birth a specialist obstetrician will separate the placenta from your uterus under anaesthetic. In a future pregnancy, you will not necessarily have a placenta accreta again, but there is an increased risk.

Placenta praevia

A placenta praevia or 'low lying' placenta has embedded in the lower part of your uterus. This is common in early pregnancy but by week 32 fewer than 1:100 women have placenta praevia. The most common symptom is on-and-off *bleeding* without pain: usually after week 30. Even if you experience some bleeding, placental function is probably normal: there is little risk to your baby. The risk is to you, with a danger of haemorrhage. Heavy bleeding around week 20 carries the highest risk. You will be advised to rest. Take vitamins and minerals suitable for pregnancy to prevent or reduce anaemia. Your baby will need to be born by caesarean because there is a risk of dangerous bleeding as your cervix dilates. If you are bleeding, you may be asked to stay in hospital until birth.

Placental abruption

With placental abruption, the placenta separates from the uterine lining. This happens in fewer than 1:100 pregnancies. Minor abruption may not cause problems but a large area of separation may affect placental function and cause heavy *bleeding*. If you bleed, get in touch with your midwife immediately. If blood loss is severe, you must go to hospital: this is an emergency. **With a minor abruption,** if bleeding is light or stops and your baby is not showing signs of distress, you will be advised to rest at home. If the placenta is not functioning well, it may be best to deliver your baby early. **A major abruption** is an emergency. You will be given a drip to replace lost fluids and you may need medication to improve clotting. Beyond week 36 if you feel well and your baby is not in distress, labour may be induced. If either of you is in distress, an emergency caesarean is essential. **After birth,** you may be given extra blood-clotting factors and oxytocin to help your uterus contract efficiently. You may need a blood transfusion. You will need to rest and eat well, and continue to take vitamin and mineral supplements (including iron).

Post-traumatic stress

If you have a difficult or upsetting experience of birth, or if you experience loss or severe shock in pregnancy, there is a small risk that you may develop post-traumatic stress. You may feel resentful or angry with your care team, your baby or your partner or be highly critical of yourself, or want to give up. You may also experience infections (e.g. colds, coughs, *candida*) and digestive symptoms (such as tummy pain, *diarrhoea*). It is important to get practical help at home and to find someone to whom you can talk in confidence. This could provide an outlet for your feelings to begin emotional healing. Another aspect of healing may be to talk to professionals who were involved when you found things difficult. Occasionally medication is helpful.

Premature labour and birth

Around 5% of babies in the UK are born before week 37, i.e. prematurely. Being born early can be a challenge for a baby, with a higher risk of difficulties the earlier birth occurs. It is also a challenge for parents. Knowing the risks, you will understandably feel anxious. It may be reassuring to know that if your baby is born after week 32, prematurity usually does not carry long-term implications. The cause of premature birth is, in most cases, unknown. It is more likely with twins and a number of conditions, including vaginal infection. **Early onset of labour:** between week 34–37, if there are no signs of foetal distress, it is safe to go ahead with a vaginal birth, providing there are no indications for a caesarean. Before week 34, you will be given corticosteroid injections that stimulate your baby's lungs to mature. You may be given medication to delay contractions for 24–48 hours. **Labour and birth:** you may be very anxious and will need to draw on relaxation techniques. Your baby will be closely monitored and if there are signs of distress, a caesarean may be the safest option. Pethidine is not recommended as it could suppress your baby's breathing at birth. **After birth,** your team will be ready with paediatric care. Your baby may need help to establish breathing or may need to be given oxygen until his lungs are fully developed. He needs to be kep warm either on your chest ('kangaroo care') or in an incubator; and fed little and often. **The earlier your baby is born,** the more intensive care he is likely to need. If he is born after week 35, he may be feeding well and ready to come home after several days. If he is born earlier, or there are underlying problems, he may need to stay for longer in the neonatal intensive care unit (NICU) or special care unit (SCBU). **See also** *special care* and PROM (page 102); www.bliss.co.uk; www.pre-maturebaby.com

Rubella

Rubella is uncommon in the UK and infection in pregnancy is extremely rare. Infection before week 17 does, however, carry a risk of causing developmental problems for a baby. After week 17 there is no risk. If you are not immune, stay away from anyone you know to be infected. If you become infected, your doctor will talk to you about the implications and you may wish to see a counsellor.

Special care

Having a baby in special care is never easy. The separation can be distressing and you may be anxious, angry and sad. Parents and babies can find it difficult to bond. Neonatal nurses and doctors are usually extremely supportive. They will help you learn how to feed, touch and care for your baby. Your baby may be shocked by an early or traumatic birth, the strange environment and by tests or feeding through tubes. He will appreciate

your touch and in many special care units (SCBU) doctors and nurses devote a great deal of love and energy to each baby. Kangaroo care, where a baby is carried skin to skin by mum or dad, is becoming widespread: for a baby, it is relaxing, improves growth and supports successful feeding; for parents, it is relaxing and is a precious chance for close contact. If your baby is given intense medical care, this will be a contrast to kangaroo care. Some parents feel well supported but it is also common to feel powerless and frustrated. If you want to have a say in issues of medication and contact, you need to be proactive, and this will difficult if you are tired and shocked or do not have many chances to talk to the doctors. Do ask for information as often as you want to: the more you know, the more confidently you will be able to contribute to choices about your baby's care. Remember to take time out and to rest. It may be possible for you to stay in the hospital. **Being at home** marks the welcome beginning of living together as a family. It can, however, be stressful, more so if you need to continue close care at home (e.g. extra oxygen, feeding tubes) and if you have other children. It is important for each of you to share your thoughts and feelings and to look after yourselves. A good friend or professional counsellor may help you. Get some practical help too, particularly if your sleep is broken. Carry your baby as often as you can in a close fitting sling – the contact will make up for the isolation of the incubator.

Your child health team will provide follow-up care in the years ahead. Most babies who need special care go on to thrive but sometimes difficulties continue. Every child is unique and your team will chart your baby's development and give you advice and support as he grows.

Still birth

In the UK, around 6:1000 babies die after week 20 of pregnancy. This tragic event is shocking and upsetting. **Rarely**, there is no prior warning, but in most cases, the diagnosis is made during pregnancy and labour is then induced (see page 108). Going through labour knowing that your baby is not alive is deeply distressing. A caesarean section may be considered but involves a longer recovery time and is seldom the preferred option.

In the days before induction you will have time to process some of your feelings and prepare: it is important to consider who will be with you, and to know about pain relief options (pages 120–5). Both parents are typically devastated after a loss. For a mother the physical impact may be huge as hormones geared to nurturing and breastfeeding are present after the birth. Despite the shock, you may need to have difficult conversations as you discuss your preferences regarding a post mortem and putting your baby to rest.

A reason for still birth is often not found, but you might want to consult your specialist to investigate if you feel it would be easier to move forward. **See also** www.uk-sands.org.

Strep B

Strep B (Group B streptococcus) is a bacterial infection in the vagina affecting 1:4 women. It only sometimes causes symptoms of vaginal discharge or urinary tract infection. Routine testing is not universal, but a test is standard if labour begins prematurely or your waters break early. **In labour** or after your waters have broken, there is a risk of passing the infection to your baby, but the potential yet rare consequences (e.g. meningitis) can usually be avoided. If you go ahead with a vaginal birth it is important to have antibiotics for at least four hours before birth to minimize the risk. A few obstetricians recommend a caeasarean. **After birth,** some paediatricians recommend antibiotic treatment from birth particularly if a baby seems unwell. You may be able to request an infection test before consenting to antibiotics. In the unlikely event that your baby is infected, antibiotics tackle the infection. Homeopathy offers further support. **Rarely** symptoms may develop more than two days after birth. If your baby has a fever, vomits, has difficulty feeding, has an unusual shrill cry, goes floppy or jerks, or you notice his fontanelle bulging, call a doctor.

Swelling (oedema)

Mild swelling in pregnancy is common, usually in the ankles, feet and toes, hands and fingers. It's due to increased fluid and may be exacerbated if you are not exercising regularly, if you stand for long periods, or when it's hot. Swelling is more common with twins. Moderate swelling may be linked with high *blood pressure* so it is important to tell your midwife. **For relief,** follow the ABC (page 19) and rest with your feet propped up for at least 10–30 minutes, once or twice a day. If something you are eating leaves you feeling bloated (e.g. beans), reduce your intake. Lie on your side to sleep or to rest as this enhances kidney function. If swelling is connected to a rise in blood pressure, taking measures to bring down blood pressure should help. **Emergency action:** go to your doctor if you have a sudden increase in swelling or any pain; puffiness in your face; or if one calf is swollen, especially if it is painful (this could be a sign of very high blood pressure or deep vein thrombosis).

Toxoplasmosis

Toxoplasmosis is an infection resulting from a parasite. It is rare in pregnant women (around 2:1000). The parasite is most commonly found in raw meat, in soil and in cat faeces and may also be contracted from sheep: if you are in contact with these, it is a wise precaution to limit your contact or avoid it altogether. Wear gloves when you are gardening, cook meat thoroughly, and wash all fruit and vegetables. If you are infected there is a chance you will pass the infection to your baby. **Early in pregnancy,** infection carries a risk of affecting eye or ear development, and mildly increases the risk of *miscarriage*. **In the last three months** it carries a smaller risk. If infection is confirmed, you may have ultrasound scans to assess your baby and your specialist may offer a foetal blood test. You may value the advice of a counsellor trained in caring for parents whose babies are affected or at risk of *congenital abnormalities*.

Twins, triplets and more

Having more than one baby is often seen as a tremendous gift, and the majority of twins and their parents enjoy a healthy and happy family life. The main concern is that there are more potential stresses and difficulties: the focus here is on potential problems. In pregnancy, you are 'high-risk' and will be monitored more closely. **At birth,** many twins are born by elective caesarean. If you are keen to try a vaginal birth, you may need to shop around for necessary support. Home birth is rarely advocated. **After birth,** if your babies have been born prematurely or one or both requires special care, the days and weeks may be trying for you all. **When you are at home** you will certainly have your hands full and need extra practical help. Ask your midwife and health visitor for advice concerning feeding, whether you choose to breast- or bottle feed. **In the long term,** a lot depends on how your babies behave. Like any parents you are likely to feel tired, you may have little undisturbed time to yourselves and there may be financial strain. Keep sight of the long-view; with each month the balance tends to improve and after the first year you will probably feel the most difficult part is over (at least until they are teenagers). See also www.tamba.org.uk; www.twinsclub.co.uk.

Vaginal discharge and itching

Light or moderate white or mucousy discharge is completely normal. It tends to increase in pregnancy. You may wear panty liners to stay fresh. If you have foul smelling or cheesy discharge, perhaps with itching and stinging or vaginal sores, this is more likely to signal infection (e.g. *candida, chlamydia, herpes*): your midwife or doctor can recommend tests for an accurate diagnosis. Usually a vaginal swab is sufficient but a blood test may be needed. You are then more likely to receive the correct treatment. **In late pregnancy,** a clear watery discharge may be amniotic fluid (see PROM, page 102). **To help,** follow the ABC (page 19) to boost your wellbeing, and specific advice depending on the infection. Continue drinking eight glasses of water a day, even though it may be uncomfortable to pee. Pouring luke-warm water over your vagina as you urinate can reduce stinging.

Vaginal tears

Many women worry that they will tear during birth. It is seldom as scary as it sounds and you will not feel the tearing if it happens. Healing is usually complete; only rarely scar tissue may give pain in the long term. Tearing does not increase urinary *incontinence*. You can take measures (pelvic floor exercises, page 81; perineal massage, page 103) to reduce the risk, but there's no guarantee. **During birth,** being upright and supported (page 118) reduces the risk of tearing. The most common tear is along the perineum between vagina and anus; occasionally a tear involves the front of the labia towards the clitoris. Tears are usually superficial (first degree) but if the underlying muscles are involved, it is second-degree. First-degree tears heal spontaneously and often do not require stitching, second-degree tears usually need to be stitched. **In labour,** if you require an episiotomy there is still a small chance that you will tear: having an episiotomy to reduce the risk of tearing is not generally recommended. **Aftercare:** if you need stitching, your midwife or obstetrician will do this under local anaesthetic while you greet your baby. The stitches will dissolve within 14 days. For relief from soreness, sit on a cushion or a rubber ring and when you pee, try pouring luke-warm water over your labia to reduce stinging. As soon as you can feel the area, begin pelvic floor exercises to encourage healing. Your midwife will check you in the weeks after birth. Homeopathic Arnica helps to reduce bruising and swelling; Hypericum is excellent for nerve and tissue damage; Bellis Perennis for deep tears. Calendula, as a tincture in the bath or soaked with water into a sanitary towel, helps healing. If you feel violated or upset by what happened, it may help to talk to a counsellor or to your midwife; such feelings may affect your approach to sex as well as your femininity and confidence in the future. **Rare event:** a tear may extend backwards into the anus and sphincter. This is a third-degree tear that requires stitching in theatre and follow-up consultations.

Varicose veins

Prominent veins are completely normal because of extra fluid. A vein is varicose when the valves in the wall lose their strength and cannot stop the back flow of blood: the vein will bulge. **In pregnancy,** varicose veins are most common in the labia (which always disappear after birth) and in the legs (where they may persist). **For relief,** follow the ABC (page 19). Sit for an hour or two each day with your feet higher than your uterus and at night try raising the foot of your bed a little. If the varicosities are in your legs, wear support tights, including during labour or a caesarean. Gentle massage with upward strokes, using olive or almond oil mixed with lemon essential oil, is often relieving. Never massage directly onto the vein. The number one homeopathic remedy is Hammelis. For

persistent or very painful varicose veins, surgery may be necessary a few months after birth. **Emergency action:** if your varicose veins throb very painfully and the pain does not reduce when you rest, and especially if you are breathless, see your doctor; these may be symptoms of deep vein thrombosis.

Vitamin K

Vitamin K is needed by the liver to make proteins that help blood to clot. At birth a baby has very little vitamin K so there is a risk of dangerous bleeding: if there is bleeding into the brain, this may cause severe problems or even death. This is rare but since giving vitamin K after birth became routine in several countries, bleeding has greatly reduced. There have been some concerns about links between a vitamin K injection and skin disorders or leukaemia, but most of these have not been substantiated. Check your hospital's policy: few hospitals routinely give an injection. Most recommend oral vitamin K in three doses (at birth, at one week and at four–six weeks) and prefer to reserve the injection for babies known to be at high risk. If you are bottle feeding your baby, just one oral dose may be recommended because formula contains added vitamin K. There may be an option for you to take vitamin K while you breastfeed, although this delivers lower amounts to your baby, you need to discuss it with your doctor. **See also** www.womens-health.co.uk/vitk.asp.

Websites

www.aims.org.uk Association for Improvements in Maternity Services, official website. Information on your own rights around pregnancy and labour care, including home birth and water birth. The emphasis is on natural birth and making a stand for your choice – which may not be necessary if you already feel well supported.

www.altonweb.com/cs/downsyndrome/index.htm Provides support and information for parents of children with Down's syndrome.

www.babyworld.co.uk Jam-packed full of information, things to buy and chances to link up with other expectant parents. Includes an online antenatal club.

www.birthchoiceuk.com A site aimed to help you make an informed choice about where you plan to give birth. Includes statistics on unassisted/instrumental/caesarean births listed by hospital and tips on home birth; plus information on birth practice, intervention, breastfeeding and more.

www.birthlight.com A lovely site encouraging relaxation and contact with your baby and gentle preparation for birth. The focus is on yoga and breathing and there is information on swimming antenatal exercise. There's also postnatal information.

www.bliss.org.uk The leading site for parents whose babies are born prematurely. Lots of information about coping in hospital, what to do at home, breastfeeding and other practicalities, personal stories and contact details for support centres across the UK.

www.depression-in-pregnancy.org.uk Bravely addresses the taboo subject of depression. Not easy to navigate, and the information is quite dense, but if you feel down you may find a lot of support here.

www.ethosbaby.com Natural products for cleaning your baby, plus environmentally sensitive nappies, bedding and clothes.

www.fathersdirect.com One of few websites devoted to men. Most of the information relates to what happens after the birth, but there are useful tips for what to expect in pregnancy, and how to prepare for birth.

www.forparentsbyparents.com Light and informal, a good place to go if you want personal stories. Not in-depth but full of links to follow to other sites.

www.funmum.com Online catalogue of maternity clothes for all occasions – worth a peek.

www.thegoodbirth.co.uk A site for birth pool hire and props like birth balls.

www.infochoice.org An excellent site supported by the Royal College of Midwives and the National Childbirth Trust, with a range of online leaflets on all the major choices you'll be faced with, including care in pregnancy and what happens during labour. Combines the latest research evidence with sensitive midwifery: it's all about informed choice. You can order a pack of printed leaflets from the site, or have them emailed to you.

www.jeyarani.com A site developed by Dr Gowri Motha, author of Gentle Birth Method, with guidance and advice on how to enjoy a gentle, peaceful pregnancy and birth by using pregnancy as an opportunity to become 'birthfit'. Tips on exercise, visualization, nutrition, detox, emotional preparation, alternative therapies and self-hypnosis are given for pregnancy and for birth. The advice remains useful even if you need a caesarean.

www.kangaroomothercare.com A website recommending carrying your baby skin-to-skin, whether she is full term or premature. The site lists research and stories that show how incredibly beneficial this is for babies and parents alike.

www.littlepossums.co.uk The UK Baby Sling Specialists – slings and papooses for your baby, plus backpacks for later.

www.mothersbliss.co.uk Comprehensive site with information on pregnancy, pre-pregnancy and your baby's first year. Quite heavily weighted towards selling products, but you may find some useful (like baby equipment and books).

www.seraphine.com Rather smart maternity and baby-wear website, worth a look if only for the delicious lingerie. Go on, treat yourself.

Books
Alternative Therapies for Pregnancy and Birth, Pat Thomas (Vega) A thoughtful and thought-provoking look at how to care for yourself through pregnancy, and what choices to make around childbirth. The book is definitely pro alternative therapies but does consider conditions that may require medical care. Dares to look at deeper issues, such as spirituality, pain and sex, in detail.

The Best Friends' Guide to Pregnancy, Vicki Iovine (Simon & Schuster) Does what it says, with heartfelt, humorous and down to earth advice on what it really can be like to be

pregnant. Not everyone's best friend talks like this, but if it feels good for you, it could be a constant bedside companion for nine months or more.

Birth and Beyond, Yehudi Gordon (Ebury Press) Britain's leading obstetrician on the journey from conception until nine months after your baby's birth, from the parents' and baby's points of view. Full of practical advice and gentle guidance, with information on baby development, lifestyle, integrated healthcare options (medical and complementary), relationships, exercise, nutrition and more, plus a detailed health guide.

Birth and Breastfeeding, Michel Odent (Clairview Books) Impassioned words from a renowned obstetrician in support of gentle birth. Using years of experience, centuries of acquired wisdom and the latest scientific information, Odent stresses the value of loving support, privacy and gentle care in pregnancy, birth and breastfeeding. He celebrates birth as the most important event in life and with this book strives to help men and women welcome their babies in the best possible way.

Birth without Violence, Frédérick Leboyer (Healing Arts Press) Poetic, moving, thought provoking and beautifully illustrated. A classic for every expectant parent: to be read in a peaceful, comfortable place as you lose yourself in the journey of birth.

Childbirth without Fear, Grantly Dick-Read (Pinter & Martin) A classic text looking at fear, conditioning, choice, love, courage, nature, faith and power. A little dated in style but the issues it addresses are as important for mothers, fathers and babies as they were when the book was first published in 1959.

Dads: Because Bringing Up Kids Ain't Hard, Mal Peachey (Cassell) Light hearted but poignant and very practical reality guide for men before and after the birth. The colour presentation and jokes may become irksome after a while, but a great book to have to hand.

From Here to Maternity, Mel Giedroyc (Ebury Press) If you want a giggle, this is the book to read. Snap shots into Mel's real-life pregnancy and lots of other things going on in her life at the time.

Gentle Birth Method, Dr Gowri Motha & Karen Swan Macleod (Thorsons) Month-by-month guidance on caring for yourself and your baby through pregnancy with suggestions for therapies, food, exercise and visualizations, and how to cope with symptoms and problems. The emphasis is on gentle and the programme is based on years of experience and the satisfaction of hundreds of women.

Going it Alone, Natascha Mirosch (New Holland) Peppered with personal stories, this book for women who aren't with their partners doesn't shirk reality and gives lots of tips and encouragement. Uplifting, reassuring and very real. It also has good general medical advice.

Making Birth Easier, Andrea Robertson (Allen & Unwin) The guide for an expectant dad and/or chosen birth partner to read in pregnancy and in preparation for birth. Reading this may help to make birth easier for you and for the woman and baby you are supporting.

New Active Birth, Janet Balaskas (Thorsons) The definitive book on natural childbirth with details on making the most of your child-bearing physiology, using yoga to tone up in pregnancy and to be stable and active in labour, and caring for yourself beyond.

Pre-parenting, Thomas R Verny & Pamela Weintraub (Simon & Schuster) Looking at babies' amazing development and sensitivity before birth, this book invites you to connect with, understand and nurture your baby through pregnancy. It also helps you to consider any issues that are difficult for you, which may range from work or money dilemmas to stress, anxiety and relationship conflict. The science is fascinating if you like the detail and there are stories too.

What should I feed my baby?, Suzannah Oliver (Weidenfeld & Nicholson) Although only the beginning of this book is dedicated to breast and bottle, the information surrounding general nutrition, what food contains, junk food, organic and happy meal times is great in pregnancy and beyond. You'll keep it with you as you wean your baby and for years to come. Recipes and menu suggestions included.

Magazines
Pick a magazine whose flavour suits you – apart from the articles they are great for doctor and midwife facts, questions and answers, recommended stockists and polls on essential equipment (prams, etc.), ideas for pregnancy, nursery and beyond, and links to all sorts of books, websites and other sources of information. There are many out there: this is the cream:
FQ (for dads)
Junior Pregnancy and Baby
Mother and Baby
Pregnancy

Index

Index

Acknowledgments

This book is built on a foundation of exploration and observation that has grown over several years. Naturally, having my own children is pivotal to this, and I thank you both for teaching me so much. Working alongside Dr Yehudi Gordon, with whom I wrote *Birth and Beyond*, has also been central – thank you for guidance and friendship, for supporting me in this project and giving obstetric advice. I'd also like to thank Dr Andy Raffles, who has given paediatric advice for this book, Felicity Fine, Kitty Hagenbach and many others from the remarkable integrated healthcare centre Viveka in London, including Dr Gowri Motha, Ann Herreboudt, Kelvin Heard and Barbara Moss. Thanks to Rachel Foux for our entertaining conversations about sex; and Bill Smith for wonderful scan pictures and insight into the ultrasound world. Closer to home, thank you Sarah for compassionate midwifery advice and for checking text; Paula for midwife tips and lending me books; Alex for paediatric insight; Linda for yoga; Don and Ang for helping me to balance family and writing; Chrissie, Jo, Emma, Andy, Mara, Kevin, Cassie for good times; and Fran for keeping me afloat. Thanks, too, to everyone who has shared stories with me. I haven't quoted everything but all the stories have filtered into the text in some way: Tim, Lisa, Mike, Jen, Sarah, John, Kenia, Gabi, Paul, Jem, Becca, Dorcas, Mum, Suzie, Beena, Fatimah, Sari, Sarah, Ben, Kyle, Sam and others. At Harper Collins, thank you Denise for getting the book off the ground; Helen for warm welcomes and calmly overseeing the whole project; Laura for painstaking work on the pictures; Bob for design and Amanda for illustrations; and Emma, thank you, it is a real pleasure to have you edit my words. Last, but certainly most, thank you Gabi for being you, and Dee, for your love in every area of my life.